Copyright © 2023 Alyssa Sherlock

All rights reserved. No part of this book may be reproduced in any form by an electronic or mechanical means, including information storage and retrieval systems, without permission in writing from the publisher, except by a reviewer who may quote brief passages in a review.

Scripture quotations taken from The Holy Bible, New International Version® NIV® Copyright © 1973 1978 1984 2011 by Biblica, Inc. TM. Used by permission. All rights reserved worldwide.

This is a work of creative nonfiction. The events portrayed are presented to the best of the author's memory and records. Some parts may have been fictionalized in varying degrees, for various purposes.

Contributor works used by permission.

First edition 2023

Editor: Kyla Neufeld

Illustrator: Amber Wallin

Designer: Amber Wallin

Contributors: Erin Toews, Amelia Warkentin

Beta Readers: Erin Toews, Tavia McKinnon, Jenny Kelson, Emily Stobbe-Wiebe

ISBN 978-1-7779181-0-1

this is a love story

poems and essays on friendship, love, and mental health

by alyssa sherlock

illustrated by amber wallin

Published by Alyssa Sherlock

Winnipeg, Manitoba, Treaty 1 Territory, Canada

www.alyssasherlock.com

for grandma

everything, always

also, for everyone who hides to protect themselves

and to everyone who has shown me how freeing it is to live bravely and openly in the light

This book discusses the topics of mental health and illness, anxiety, depression, eating disorders, and suicidal thoughts. Please take care of yourself as you read.

I am grateful to live on the ancestral lands of Treaty 1 Territory and the homeland of the Métis people. I acknowledge that my water is sourced from Shoal Lake 40 First Nation.

did you know

i spend my time

writing love letters

to days

to places

to this life

did you know

this is a love letter

to you

table of contents

nim 2

anxiety 8

is this the wind 14

perfect 18

afraid 19

daily thoughts 21

make me someone else 20

(why do you write like you're) running out of time 23

my friend ED 26

my mom is sick 29

my mom is sick (ii) 30

saviour complex 31

space 32

love 34

let go 35

ode to a cinnamon bun 36

depression 38

depression translations 52

fix 53

monster 55

recovery 55

these little things 59

rest 62

impaction (life jumping) 63

the process of self-love 65

restoration	67
twins: 15 months apart	68
how to measure friendship	71
chicago (with you)	73
the faith of the matriarch	74
dear grandma	78
heartbreak	81
forgive	84
grown up	85
waves	86
kindred spirits	88
tilt-a-whirl	96
what really happened in Vancouver	97
long distance	97
winter song	97
served with love	97
desert girl in prairie summer storm	97
here's where i fell in love	97
friday night	97
resources that helped me	97
acknowledgments	97
about the author	97

nim

    I sit at a table, my hands in my lap. My body quivers with nerves and excitement. Five other friends surround me, their own knowing smirks on their faces, ready with their secrets. The scene is set. I take a mouthful of popcorn, fiddle with my new dice. New voices spill from my mouth, and my friends', and soon after a waterfall of laughter follows. Everything on this night is electric. I'm consumed, enraptured. Slowly, thoroughly, I disappear.

～ɾɹ℮

    There was once a wood elf named Nim. She grew up deep in the forests of Iry, where green brush darkens the sky, in an isolated clan of other wood elves. The branches of the thick trees would curl around the elves and protect them from the outside world, but Nim didn't mind. She had her family, her mom and her little sister and her little brother, and her best friend Thea, and that was enough for her. She would do anything for the people she loved. Sometimes, as she and Thea spent time falling into misadventures and wandering just a bit too far off the path, Nim wondered about her father, a figure that had been absent her entire life. But really, he was no one that truly mattered.

    She also had a secret.

    Nim's clan of wood elves was known for their isolation and their distrust of the other. Some of those strange creatures they looked down upon were the Ents, trees that spoke and lived and maybe loved, but mostly kept to themselves. This wood elf clan, however, hated Ents, for their passivity and aberration of nature. Trees, the clan chief proclaimed, were meant to be trees, not humanoid creatures that breathed.

    Nim knew the hatred of Ents well; it was ingratiated into her very skin. It was the only thing her absent father had left behind: her arms were bark, her fingers branches; her legs thick, rough trunks exactly like the trees that surrounded her every day. She covered them up with long, wide-legged pants, long sleeves, and white gloves that she never, ever took off. Her mother reassured Nim and her other half-tree siblings that they were beautiful and unique and had nothing to be ashamed of, even as she pleaded with them, for their own safety, to stay hidden.

Then Nim let her secret out, just a crack. But the crack was enough to let a flood burst forth, and suddenly the whole clan knew of their Ent heritage. Nim and her family stood before the clan chief, who banished them from the forest for being abominations to nature. Nim was filled with hatred, mostly at herself for being so trusting. She had known all along that she was hated, would be hated, if she ever shared too much of herself. And she had gone and shared too much of herself anyway. She had learned her lesson. She would never open up like that again; she would bury the bark on her skin deep.

Nim and her family found themselves in a world they'd never known: a dry, cracked desert wasteland of a city. Nim and her family now lived in a city slum, where people subsisted on close to nothing. Nim watched as her family withered, getting sicker and sicker with every passing day they spent away from the forest. Nim, desperately searching for answers and solutions, found herself at the temple of a nature god, hoping that she could somehow restore her family to health. The god helped her some, and she gained some power from them, but they could only do so much. The only thing Nim ever wanted to do was protect her family. So, in order to save them, she left. She had only ever known the desert city slums and the isolated forest, so she hired a guard to lead her to new places.

Along the way, though—in a small tavern in a town that was so small as to almost not be a town—some sort of weird black mist attacked, and suddenly Nim found herself travelling with a group of strangers, including the guard she had first hired to help her begin her journey. She told herself it was for protection, that she could make use of their astounding power, even as deep down, she knew she liked the company. Over the next few weeks-turned-months, she found herself becoming fond of this ragtag group of misfits, as much as she kept her walls up, while they teased her about her abrasiveness. Through little moments—the gift of a longbow, conversations on nighttime watches—Nim slowly softened, although her skin was definitely still made of bark.

Slowly, she started to wonder what would happen if she revealed herself fully. Maybe it would be okay. Maybe they would accept her, even love her, just as she was. Sometimes, when she showed a bit of herself, her companions joked that she did have a mushy inside despite her gruff exterior. When the party came across a monstrous tree, a few of her companions noted the similarities between Nim and the tree, eventually drawing the incorrect conclusion that wood elves and trees were one and the same. While Nim corrected the assumption, she couldn't help but wonder what would happen if they knew how close they were to the truth.

Their adventures continued, and the intrigue got deeper, and soon the things Nim and her friends—they were friends now—were dealing with got bigger. Their problems were as big as the world, and they were somehow supposed to stop the end of it. Nim's secrets, and her struggle over revealing them, fell to the background. There were plenty of opportunities for Nim to come clean, but she used none of them. It was safer to stay hidden. And then it was time to defeat the evil they had fought for so long to uncover. They spent hours hatching a plan, and, finally, they were ready to defeat their enemy.

And then everything just… stopped.

Nim was my Dungeons & Dragons character. Dungeons & Dragons is a collaborative storytelling tabletop role-playing game that I started playing with my brother, some friends, and friends of friends the summer of 2018. Nim was my first character. I created her over the course of six months while we prepared for our first campaign—a long, connected, running story played in multiple weekly sessions over the course of months or years. We played that campaign for almost two years, moving online and to weekly once the pandemic of 2020 began. It's joked about in D&D circles that your first character (if you like to delve deep into backstory and character development like I do) is basically just you under a thin layer of fantasy game mechanics. Nim is me in many ways. Over the course of years of playing her and rationalizing her actions and decisions, I learned a lot about myself too. I learned about my pride and my distrust of others, my judgmental nature, and my uncertainty about taking the reins of leadership even when I was best suited to that role. I also learned about my own tendency to hide things, because it was so much safer to not reveal myself or be vulnerable.

Throughout the campaign, I waited for the moment when Nim would be "found out," the moment that something would happen that would reveal her true Ent features to the party, whether she wanted to or not. That never happened.

My brother (and our Dungeon Master, the one who runs the game and corrals the party of players) called me out on it, saying I could just bring it up myself if I wanted to. But I didn't want to have to do that.

So I waited.

And then the campaign ended abruptly, with a promise to end our final fight once we could play safely in person again. As of this writing, that time hasn't come, and our memories of the intrigue and connective threads of that story dim with every passing day. I realized I should've just done it: let Nim reveal her own secrets. How amazing would that moment have been? Nim hadn't shared because she was stubborn and scared, and now she would never get that beautiful (and probably hilarious) moment of connection from revealing herself.

Just like me.

This book is me, taking off my gloves, rolling up my sleeves, and showing you the rough, rough bark underneath.

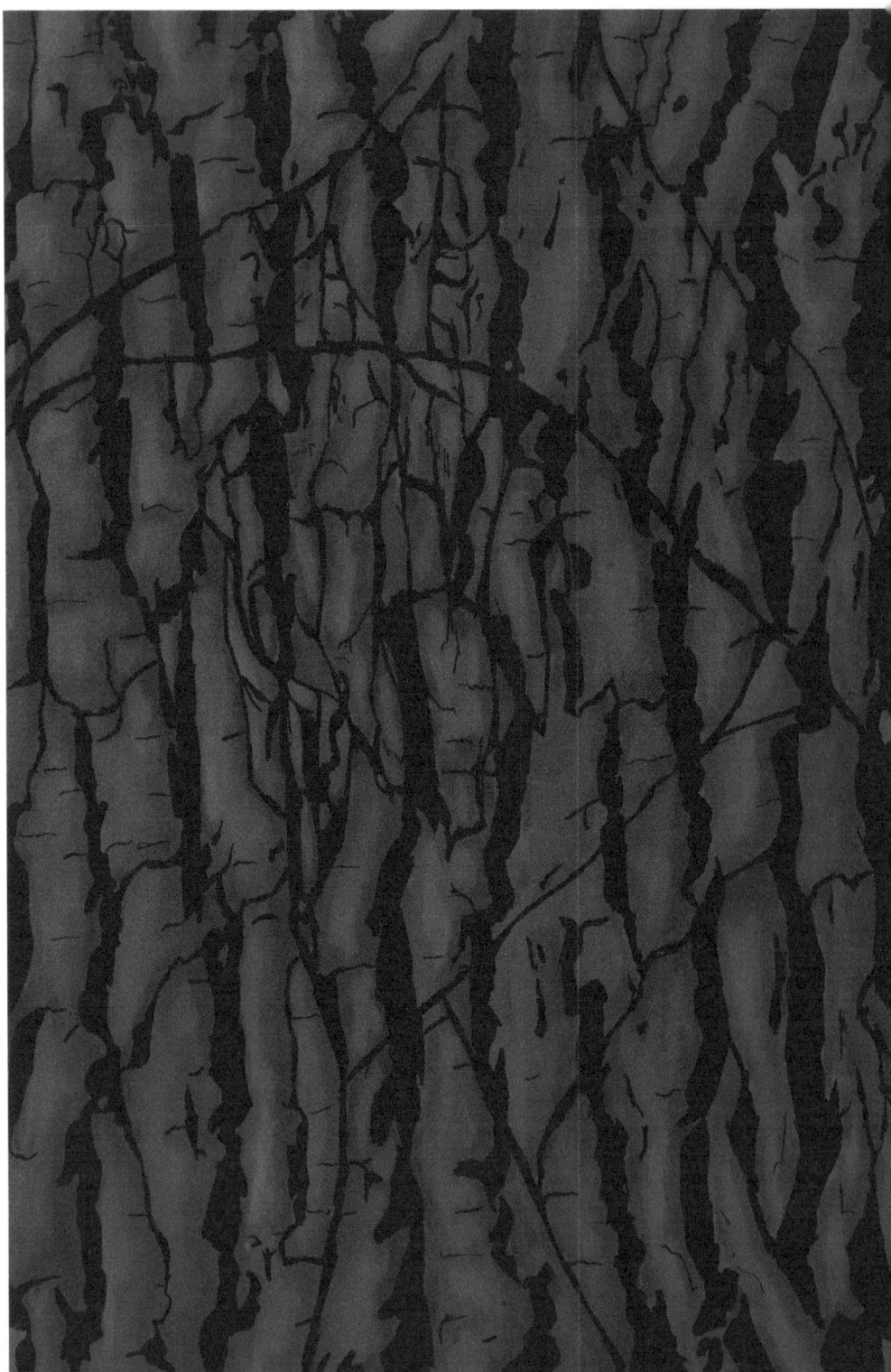

anxiety

I stand beneath a trellis at the back of the field where my cousins' wedding ceremony is going to happen in just a few moments. I stand amidst the legs of the adults fussing around me. My heart races, and my stomach flip flops over itself. I grip the basket of fake petals that I'm to litter the aisle with in just a few moments. The adults fuss over my little flower girl crown. It's an incredible amount of responsibility, and I can't quite take it. Up come the contents of my stomach, thankfully not much but a clear bile that doesn't leave a mark on my white lace dress.

I sit in the bathtub and cry while my mom washes my hair and listens patiently. The lunch monitor at school was mean again. My sensitive heart can't take the strict, no-nonsense harshness of a lunch monitor trying to control hordes of rowdy kids let loose. I take every scolding that is meant for troublemakers on my own shoulders, even as I sit meekly and silently eating my lunch. I have nightmares about the lunch lady, her short dark hair monstrous in the darkness of night, her barks louder and more menacing. Mom slips a Bible verse into my lunch kit: "For I am the Lord your God who takes hold of your right hand and says to you, Do not fear; I will help you" (Isaiah 41:13, NIV). I fold up the slip and repeat the verse to myself over and over again in a trance when I am afraid. I remember the verse years later, always holding it close in panic-filled moments.

I start a new school. I'm separated from my best friend. Weird things are happening to my body, and my mom is sick a lot, on and off. Everything is scary. I don't want to go to school. When I have to go to school or choir concerts, I lock myself in my room and scream and cry, yelling that I'm certain bad things are going to happen to me if I go. My mind is certain of the terrors that await me. Eventually my parents are able to push me out of the house. When we get home, they say, "See, that wasn't so bad, was it?"

I don't want to do anything. I hide under my covers and play on my Game Boy for hours, attempting to block out the scary world around me.

I look at my cat, curled up by the heating vent, and wish with a physical ache that I could be him. No worries, no responsibilities—just sleep, eat, and be taken care of. I lie in bed and hold my breath, hoping I can hold it long enough to disappear from this terrifying world. My parents take me to the doctor to see if I'm depressed. The doctor concludes I'm not, and that's that. I still don't know what's wrong with me, but somehow the spiral slows as I open myself up to my friends at church youth group, start to pray, and find someone else out there is in control and taking care of me. I develop some coping mechanisms. I start to feel a bit less afraid.

I get a new job, one of my first "real" jobs, with a biweekly paycheque and clocking in and out. It's my first day. My heart races, my palms sweat, and my breath comes quicker. My mind gets stuck on little things—where do I go when I first get there? What if someone points out I don't belong? What if I made a mistake and wasn't actually hired like I thought I was? The door is locked when I arrive, and it's the end of the world. Now I'm late, and they're going to know I'm a mistake. They tell me I should be here before they open. I don't mention I didn't know there was a doorbell to call someone. I already feel terrible for making such a stupid mistake.

It's my fifth year of university. I should feel like I know things now. I've written so many papers, I've done group projects good and bad, I know where all my classes are, I know the culture. I know that you sit in the chapel lounge to wait for class and the north campus lounges for a quiet place to nap or study. My brain fills with what ifs, the most prominent, *what if NOW is the moment when everything goes wrong?* I arrive an hour early for a new class and ask the building receptionist where the class is. He shows me and opens the classroom for me. Objectively, it's no big deal, but it's not the case in my mind. My heart beats wildly and my chest feels tight and my limbs all quivery. It wears me down with questions and accusations. *I'm such a loser, I just asked the receptionist where the class was?? I'm an hour early?? I should have taken a later bus. Maybe I should go to the student lounge? But I just said I was fine here to that guy; what will he think if I go upstairs? Okay, I'll go upstairs... I'm pretty sure everyone is staring at me. They know I don't know what I'm doing. How long should I wait before going back to the classroom? What is the least awkward time to show up in class? Great, now I'm late and there's like five spots left, and oh no I have to sit near the front...*

I'm crushed by the weight of the world. My thoughts race fastest at night. They're impossible to block out through headphones or counting numbers backwards. My mind leaps, tumbles, spins from one thought to the next, picking up speed as it runs away downhill. I worry about not being able to sleep. In the morning, I'm paralyzed, my body frozen. I'm certain I'm dying.

I sit at my desk and shake. My head, my fingers, my toes all tingle and buzz like a horde of ants have taken over and buried into my skin. I scratch at my shoulders with my nails, trying to get them out. My skin bleeds. I'm running out of time, and it's always too late, and I haven't done enough. I'm on the precipice of death. Everything, every little mistake, even as minuscule as forgetting my phone at home, is death or the end of the world. I can't focus because there's too much to do, too much to think, and, no matter what I do, I'm certain I'll do it wrong, so I don't do it. My heart races, my stomach flops, I gag and retch. I can't catch my breath.

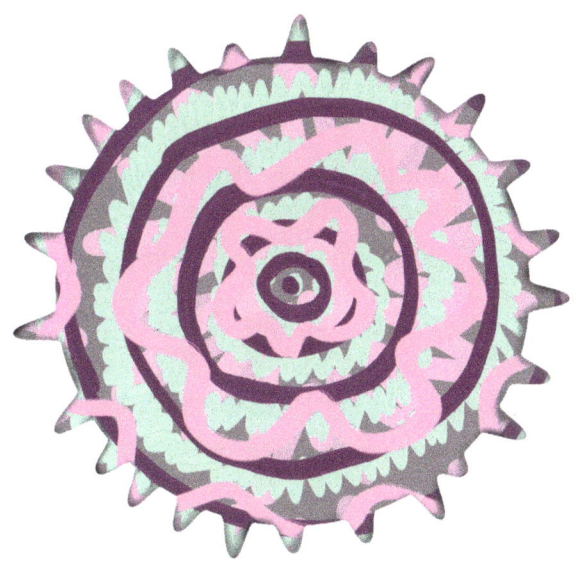

I can't sit still. I get up. I feel trapped in the room. I walk down the hallway. I feel trapped there too. Outside, I'm trapped. I'm trapped in my own mind. It spins and spins and spins and rolls away from me. I want to tear my skin off, violently scratch out this brain that's intent on attacking me and keeping me hostage with overwhelming fear and spinning, spiralling thoughts. *What if what if what if what if?* What if my parents die? What if I die? What if everything I've ever believed—like that people love me and care about me—is actually not true and I've been making it up this whole time? I live in the future, in every possibility, all of them awful. Everything bad will happen to me and every good thing *will* end. My mind is stuck on the worst outcome. Anything can happen to anyone. Anything can happen to me.

me

Over the years, my anxiety has slowly become a companion, something that annoys and frustrates me, but that I've kind of learned to live with. I didn't actually have a name for the feeling until after high school, thanks to the internet and various media I consumed, made by young, anxious women like me. The thing I felt was called *anxiety*, and not everyone felt it. It actually wasn't normal to be afraid of almost everything, all of the time. Not everyone thinks death is a certain outcome when they do something new, or finds it much more difficult to do basic, seemingly easy tasks. It's a struggle to realize that your own brain is making your life much more difficult than it needs to be, especially when people don't believe you or think it's not a big deal because "everyone gets anxious sometimes." If I've learned anything from my liberal arts education, it's that naming is powerful. Giving my anxiety a name helped me separate out those irrational feelings and fears from more rational ones, even if I didn't always do it right.

At best, anxiety for me is a constant barrage of questions and accusations, an overthinking of every minuscule aspect of life. At worst, it's the precipice of death. It's a constant, exhausting battle. Sometimes, anxiety is my companion, a unique way of looking at the world that gives me empathy and compassion, makes me pause and go slower to analyze, see details, and be thorough—but, only sometimes. While I value being careful, more often than not, my desire for going slow and picking out details comes from a fear of being wrong. Other times, anxiety is my enemy. It keeps me in place out of fear, enabling me to run away, escape and hide from hurt, but also joy. If I could, would I choose this? No, probably not. It sucks. I hate it and just want to live a normal, carefree life like everyone else. But, it's also a part of me, and I don't know who I'd be without it.

is this the wind

is this the wind
terrible, buffeting rage
screaming through
open sky too wide

are these the trees
creaking and moaning
holding together the cracks
between the earth

is this my mind
a thundering avalanche
crushing soundlessly
burying alive

is this me
earth eroding
crumbling away
leaving roots exposed

and does it
have to be?

perfect

I was always a straight-A student. In the fourth grade, my parents put me in the GATE program. I can't remember the full acronym now, but I know the "G" stood for "Gifted." Being in GATE meant that every so often my other "gifted" friends and I got to spend a class separated from our idiotic, troublemaker classmates to do things like make up our own board games from scratch. I thrived on the approval of teachers and the hope that, if I did everything right, I would get top marks.

In high school, I went into the International Baccalaureate program, the advanced program for more academically-serious students. I measured my marks against my friends'. If a friend was upset with a 98%, then I was definitely devastated by my measly 90%. Still, school and academics came relatively easy to me. I knew how to meet the strict expectations placed upon me. There was a system with right and wrong answers, and all I had to do was figure out the right answer to succeed. Even in university, where discussions became more abstract and nuanced, and where I delved with my professors and classmates into global social justice issues with no easy answers, we still had to put all our learnings to paper for a nicely quantifiable grade. Life was easier when it was measurable, when there were obvious right and wrong answers, and I held onto this as a lifeboat when emotions, anxiety, and uncertainty swirled around me.

I'm a perfectionist, but being a perfectionist is far from the quirky, detail-oriented stereotype people often talk about. It's said as a fun, cheeky answer to the interview question, "what is your weakness?" It's not that, though. It's actually an insidious belief that if you do nothing wrong, if you make no mistake, you can protect yourself from failing or being hurt.

But that doesn't work, because perfection is impossible. Though we attempt to avoid failure by being perfect, in reality perfectionism causes failure because perfection does not exist. I can't be the perfect daughter, the perfect sibling, the perfect roommate, the perfect friend, the perfect employee—every slip, every mistake, is another reason I'm not good enough. Slowly, they stack up to the point of overwhelming self-hatred.

The structure of academics is familiar and safe. If only there were a grading rubric for life. Then I could know exactly how to move forward into the unknown. That's not to say I haven't tried to create my own life rubric, grasping at societal rules or my own personal convictions to create a grading structure for myself, for my relationships, for my work, and for every aspect of my life. If I structure my life enough, I can eliminate the terrifying grey, the nuance and uncertainty that often unhinges me. I must grip onto something concrete, because it is terrifying when there is too much out of my control.

I'm a hostage to perfection. I'm afraid to make a move, get messy, and expose myself for fear of being less than, of messing up, of hurting myself or others. I used to look down my nose at those that plowed ahead messily, not slowing down enough to pay attention and plan ahead to prevent mistakes. Now I envy them, forging ahead with abandon, being messily vulnerable, getting stuff done even as they constantly stumble through. They are free.

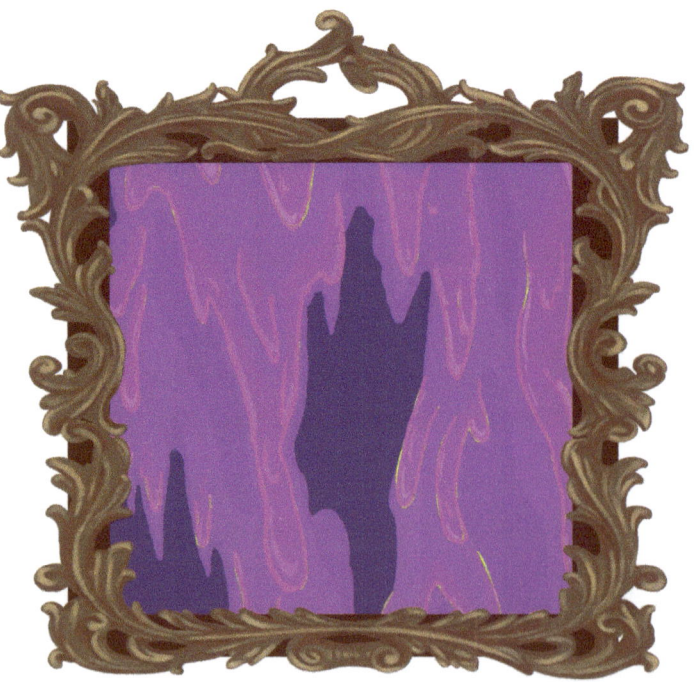

afraid

shallow breaths fight the deep open sky
heart beats wildly, not steady enough
to stand firm against the wind

this high up, logic is a liar
there are no railings on top of the world
and everything is terrifyingly exposed

my stomach drops into the blue
and all that remains
are endless possibilities for falling

daily thoughts

i'm useless
i should be talking more
leave the comfort zone
why should i
did she really just say that
i'm right
do i know anything
am i selfish? probably
too many people
i miss my friends
wish i was anywhere but here
wish i was the opposite of me
when will i learn
i love music and these walls
why did i park so far away
i'm an idiot
stop your stupid mouth
am i selfish? definitely
i can't believe i forgot
i go outside you know

make me someone else

I'm alone. The cream-yellow walls of the three-room apartment I share with my aunt and uncle seem more bare than normal tonight. My aunt and uncle are out with their friends. My family and everyone I love, who I left months ago to search for myself while volunteering at an international school in the Philippines, seem impossibly far away.

Outside in the tropical heat, students run past, laughing. Inside the apartment, the air conditioning units fill the space with recycled air and I'm trapped in a cold, empty tomb. My mind races, flipping over itself and squeezing my chest and my stomach until I can't stand it anymore and need to turn it off. I race to my computer, which is broken, but it's not an option anymore to let the buzz of silence fill my thoughts with frantic, desperate worry. I sneak up to my aunt and uncle's room and pull my aunt's computer from her backpack, quickly opening up YouTube to lose myself in the lives of other people there.

There, on the screen, are happy people, living and laughing together. For a moment, they invite me into their lives. I'm not sitting in an empty apartment by myself, but riding along for their adventures. My heart rate settles, and the world around me fades away. I'm not me anymore, I'm them, and I'm relieved. I want to be them, with their adventurous lives and smiles, even as I know, deep in the back of my mind, this isn't really them, but a slice. It doesn't matter; their world is obviously better than mine. They are more experienced, have more friends, do lots of fun jobs, and are incredibly talented. I love them for offering their connection to me. I hate them for everything they are that I'm not. I lose myself in video after video, time rolling by as my life is slowly, disastrously consumed by theirs.

Eventually, I look up from the screen, the world around me settling. I feel queasy, slightly dirty.

I'm still alone.

(why do you write like you're) running out of time

tick-a thump-a tick-a thump-a

it's coming coming *coming* **coming**

can't stop can't stop

go go go *go*

walls closing sand

filling nostrils stinging

arms flailing can't sink

can't it's coming

closer closer CLOSER

not enough time not enough t

im being left behi—

can't stop can't stop

legs aching lungs burning

can't stop coming closing

ending the end is closing in

ending ending *ending* **ending**

much too near to nevers

must be *now now now* **NOW**

run *run* **run** **R U N**

can't stop can't stop can't
can't stop can't stop can't
can't stop can't

my friend ED
Amelia Warkentin

I hike up my underwear so it lands just above the roll of fat.
Lamenting how this area used to be flat.
When hunger was my virtue.

The raging beast was contained by protruding ribs;
like bars of a cage, they exemplified "thin."
The beast consumed the spot where my heart had been.

Growls were the source of my vanity.
Louder than rumbling emptiness was my shame.
On appearance destined to falter, I now lay my blame.

Now, one bite after another.
Make it routine.
Don't overthink—suppress the scream.
The fear will go away, "they" say,
but are "they" really on my team?!

When it was just ED and me, my heart would palpitate—fly.
I could soar right through mealtimes, my energy high.
I could sleep very little, as if I'd never die.

But ED had rules.
If I didn't follow,
my life would be over—forgotten.
There would be no tomorrow.

Each day was a vacuum. It sucked motivation—
consumed me while I consumed very little.
What I thought was power, I realize was pain.
When ED had control, my thinking was inane.

My hunger was a tomb for productivity.
Yet my worth was determined by my abilities.
My friend ED was a toxic addiction.
An affair that forbade food—caused much contradiction.

Now I know it's food that allows me to survive.
If ED were still my friend, I wouldn't be alive.

my mom is sick

the door is closed
the oven cold
countertops clean and stark
an empty seat at the kitchen table
dad says it's sandwich night again

the door is closed
blocks strength i'm desperate for
no one sings away my worries
or strokes my forehead to calm me down
or untangles the twists in my thoughts

the door is closed
i bury deep beneath the covers
plug my ears to sounds of sick
shiver away until morning
wish away the unrecognizable, terrified

the door is closed
i spin a net of worries
throw a tantrum
yank at the locked doorknob
it doesn't work; the world still falls apart

my mom is sick (ii)

i give up my space as a human
indenture myself to healing

i boil myself into a balm
rub myself on your aches

i pour myself into a gel capsule
let you swallow me whole

i inhabit your skeleton
twist out the stiff joints

i dive into your acid
settle your roiling stomach

i pull down your heavy eyelids
cover your restlessness

nothing changes
so what does that make me

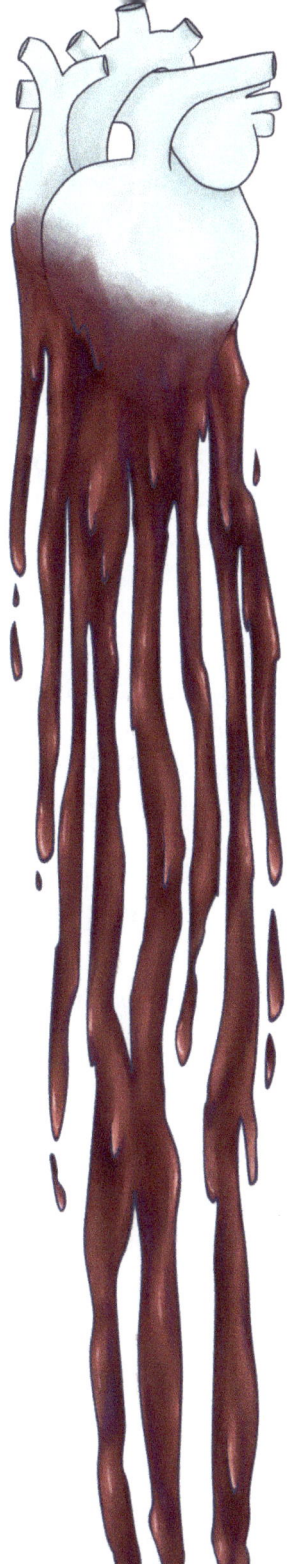

saviour complex

There's something wrong with you, and I respond promptly with a list of things you should do. Maybe you should see a therapist. Maybe you should go to church. Maybe a god would give you a sense of purpose. I have a friend who knows a thing, maybe I can connect you. I read an article; you should read it. There's a book I read exactly for your situation. I'll lend it to you.

I read everything I can, trying to understand. Google is not a great place to find answers, but maybe if I just look hard enough and use the right combination of search terms, I'll eventually find one. The perfect article, the one that gives me a direction, a concise set of steps to follow. I read and I read and I read. It's not enough.

If you can't, then I can. I am the meal-maker and the house-cleaner, and I buy cards and write letters and send gifts. I send texts and well wishes, pithy sayings that feel like nothing (I Googled what the right thing to say is). You're still sick.

I refuse to accept that there's nothing I can do, so I keep doing until my soul is exhausted. If you're weak, I'm strong; if you're a mess, then I can be put together. I'm going to be the one you need, the one who will pull you out and return you to health. I'm going to do everything. I'm going to be everything. I'm going to save you. I'm going to fix this. If I don't, what do I do? Scream. Cry.

Maybe you did this to yourself. Why can't you just be better? Why aren't you trying? Why are you lying in bed? Maybe if you just got out of bed, turned on the lights. Maybe if you ate the right diet and exercised. I can make the meals for you, force you to take care of yourself. You don't. You stay behind closed doors. I hate you. Being angry is easier than admitting helplessness. People tell me to wait, be patient, to just be there. No more doing. Sit and listen.

It feels like nothing.

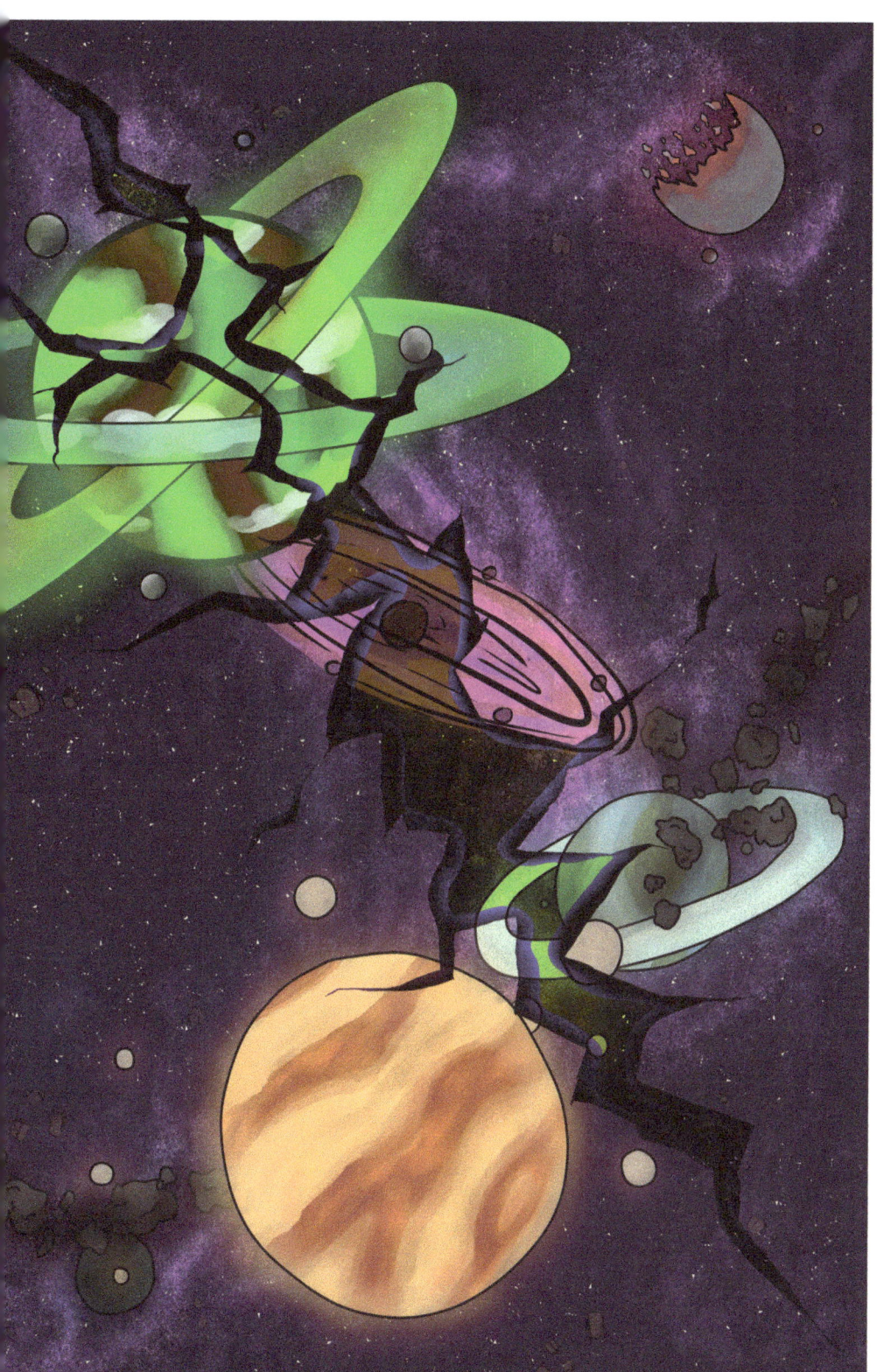

space
Erin Toews

Inside my home, we're freshly fed
with fantasy and trifle.
Michael Bublé wafts through air embossed
by long-armed lamps, whose lights are powerful
enough to shroud the night
made warm by 26 of us.
We mix and spill and laugh like liquids,
morph and flow to meet an edge.
Everyone is comfortable
but you, hunched, chin in hand.
I tilt my head to see your lowered eyes are black.
I lean forward, look through your lenses
discover you're floating in space

        your fears an infinite haze of stars you face

                          in harried glimpses endlessly twirling

    hurtling to an unknown place

            muscles stiff

                              stomach churning

                                        ears plugged

        collision bound

Where's a rope?
I'll scale my neighbour's oak
and wave and jump and shout your name.
Closer to the night you'll have to notice me.
I'll rescue you and reel you home.

But you're too far away to see
and sound can't travel there.
Shattered, I crash
onto the loveseat with our friends
and gaze out through the window pane.
The moon is fully luminous,
and, with a start, I spot your soul
float a speck across it—
not impossible, with help, to recover.

love

i thought maybe it was

fixing
tinkering with broken wires
reattaching frayed synapses

shaping
smoothing rough edges
attempting to make beautiful

fighting
screaming and begging
making you save yourself

i was wrong

it's really
wondering
stepping back
pulling desperate hands away
letting grow

let go

fingers curl
muscles strain
only my skin
keeps everything secure
nothing allowed to slip through

but this grasp is
merely an illusion
i grip onto air
while my palms ache and burn

instead
i peel these fingers back
one by one
let the emptiness fall
leave these hands open
anticipating

ode to a cinnamon bun

Amelia Warkentin

Stupid cinnamon bun. I hate you.

You take over my thoughts until I go out of my way to possess you.
But though I hold you, guilt forbids me to eat you.

I fight a battle in my mind, then all at once I succumb.

I linger in the first taste of carbs and sweetness—
the perfect blend of cinnamon and sugar on my tongue.

Tearing at my self-control, the bun takes its hold.

Still warm, succulent, simple—I return again and again.
Not wanting to stop, lamenting that I ever started.
What will I do when I'm done? It's likely I'll want another one.
And what about tomorrow: will I cave to this craving again?
Should a diet not be more than cinnamon buns?

Fears surface and scold

Questions of origin, ingenuity and "how's" flood my thoughts:
Who created such splendor, such genius, such gold?
When did I discover this weakness? Why does it never grow old?
How did this combination, these proportions, come to be?
How can a food make me tongue-tied and then fill me with glee?

Around and around I go, until I reach the end—the middle.

I'm not convinced those last bites are the best.
They're sometimes too sweet, over saturated, underwhelming.
They're the ending to an experience that I began resenting.

Darling cinnamon bun. I love you.

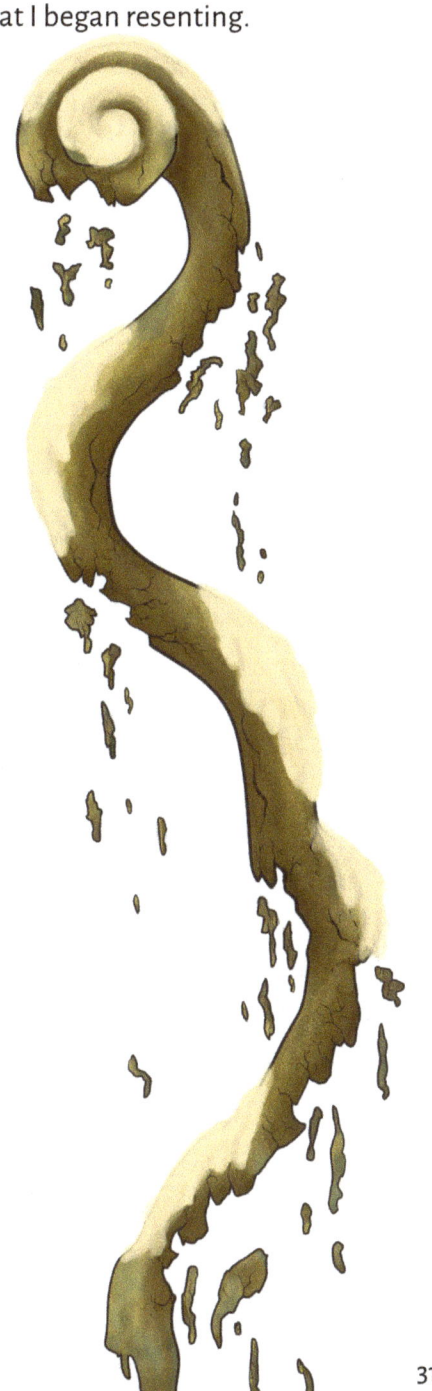

depression

I sit in a car beside my best friend, parked on the street outside her house. She's just confessed stiffly, awkwardly, that she's been diagnosed with clinical depression. The silence is full. I've always been a helper, but I'm also always concerned with making the wrong step, saying the wrong thing. I don't know what to do here. I don't really understand. I'm desperate to understand. I desperately need things to make sense.

So I write.

~me

"I have depression."

That morning, Sam had texted Mara and said that she had something important to tell her later that night. Mara had spent the entire day trying to do other things while worrying about what the thing was. It sounded serious. She had gone over every single possibility in her head. Someone was dying. Sam's mother. Or Sam was pregnant, although Mara was fairly certain Sam was still a virgin. Or she was moving out. Maybe she was moving to another country, and living in a remote hillside far away from any internet connection. That thought made Mara have to put down her book and grip the comforter beneath her, coaxing herself to get her breathing back to normal.

"Oh," was all Mara could think to say. The tension in her chest deflated a bit, because really, it wasn't as bad as she'd imagined. In all her fourteen years of knowing Sam, it actually made sense. And then at the same time, it was devastating. "I'm—" Mara started, but every word that could come after was insufficient.

Sam fidgeted with the seat belt latch, pushing the red button in and out. "Yeah."

"This doesn't change anything," Mara said, and then immediately regretted it, because she didn't know what she was talking about.

"Okay," Sam said.

"I love you," Mara said.

Sam smiled, softly and wistfully, like she was a looking across the horizon at a place that she loved, but was leaving. "I know."

They hugged, the world shifted, and Mara felt simultaneously a hundred years older and like a nervous child, uncertain of the new world opening up before her.

Mara read the entirety of the Wikipedia page and five other descriptions on medical journal sites before being disappointed that she wasn't finding the information she desperately wanted. Clinical depression was more than a bad mood. There was something about a chemical imbalance in the brain. The causes of depression were unknown. The cause was possibly trauma in youth or genetics. Then there were suicide statistics, which Mara scrolled quickly past as her heart rate sped up.

But I don't understand, Mara thought. *What does this mean for her? For me?*

She found a video of a children's book, *I Had a Black Dog* by Matthew Johnstone. It was only a few minutes long, so she watched it. The author talked about a black dog following him around, sitting on his chest, dragging him down. Some heavy, outside force, dark and crushing.

"The black dog will always be with me," said the narrator.

Mara felt utterly helpless.

Mara watched silently and noticed. Sam talked about sleeping a lot. She was always having naps. When they took the bus to school together, Sam would nap, or look tired and lost, or scroll through Facebook on her phone, especially if they saw a friend of Mara's and they talked. Mara tried not to let herself get frustrated. *Sam's sick*, she wanted to say, to explain. Thankfully people their age didn't have phone etiquette, so nobody really cared anyway that Sam would blatantly ignore them to get lost in Facebook memes.

Every day, Mara asked the same thing just before her stop. "Want to come over, study and watch a show or something?"

Sam pressed her forehead to the bus window and closed her eyes. "Nah, I'm pretty tired. Tomorrow, maybe."

She always said *tomorrow*. Mara got off the bus at her stop and watched it pull away, glimpsing the top of Sam's limp brown hair through the window. The sky was clear blue, but Mara felt grey inside. She wondered if the grey feeling was contagious, if she had caught it. She so badly wanted to do something. She couldn't say just be happy, because it wasn't that easy. She couldn't say it would get better, because she didn't know. Maybe it wouldn't get any better. She could say, *I'm here for you, I love you*, but what did that do? She could say, *The bad days don't last. Don't die on me.*

When she got home, she grabbed a book and a Coke and went to the backyard to read. She lay on her back on the grass, holding the book above her face. She stared at the pages, at the words, and they blurred, and her thoughts wandered. *There are bad days and good days*, the book said. On the bad days, you feel stuck. You feel sluggish, like you can't do anything or go anywhere. There's a force stopping you from doing life normally. You just *can't*. It's a physical inability to do life.

Mara tried to imagine it. She tried to imagine a darkness so strong and suffocating surrounding her, weighing her down, preventing her from life. She could imagine how hard it could be to push against the current, swim to the surface and gasp for air, when she couldn't even bring herself to believe there was a surface to swim to. She could imagine how people could want to escape the suffocation of life. Mara squeezed her eyes shut, dropping her book onto her chest. Remember the good days, she prayed. There are always good days.

She opened her eyes. As much as she could imagine it, she couldn't feel it. The air around her was light. The wind was cool. The sun shined.

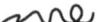

I wrote this piece the day after I sat in that car, in an effort to try to understand. As I got older, more people I knew told me they had experienced depression. I read books and dove deep into Wikipedia articles on depression, but I was still lacking a fundamental understanding. I didn't get it. I didn't really understand why the depressed members of my households stayed in bed all day. Why couldn't they at least get some chores done while the rest of us were out working all day? I was frustrated with the constantly delayed responses to texts or the tiring negativity in response to my attempts at encouragement.

I never thought it would be me. But, a tumultuous and unhealthy workplace; a pandemic; separation from coworkers, friends, and family; ever-increasing anxiety that eventually became daily, consistent panic attacks; and increasing back pain and medication that made me feel sick and out of it all the time, all made me ripe for a breakdown. I didn't notice it until the train was already reeling off the tracks.

me

I'm not going to cook this week; it's too much work. I'll do something more interesting than pasta next week. Next week comes. The cookbook stays closed. Summer's coming. Good, something to enjoy, something to look forward to. Once this stressful period at work is over, things will get better. I'm not going to do this work task, there's no point. Is responding to this email really that important in the grand scheme of things? It doesn't really matter. Nothing matters. I want to go home. Okay, I'm home now. I don't feel any better.

I go hiking on the beach with my housemates. They go to scrounge for wild blueberries in the bush, and I stay on the lakeshore by myself, surrounded by sparkling blue. All my problems, all the world's problems, are far away. I wish to stay there forever.

My limbs feel like lead. I can't sleep. The nights are long and torturous, filled with anxious thoughts. When I do sleep, I don't feel rested. I'm asleep even when awake, and someone has turned off the lights. My vision is weird, and the sky is dim. I can't open my eyes wide enough. Maybe if I exercise, I'll wake up. Maybe if I put my contacts in? Maybe if I eat something? Go for a walk? Splash my face with cold water, again and again and again? Nope. Nothing. It's a Herculean effort to get out of bed.

I dread work every moment, and weekends are only a blink of hating the passage of time before Monday. What's the point? I'm only getting up to drag myself to a job I hate, to then come home drained of energy to do anything but get ready for the next day, then suffer through a restless sleep, then repeat until the weekend, when I waste the speeding time away dreading Monday's return.

I don't have the energy to choose clothes, so I recycle the same three outfits, day after day. I've forgotten how to dress. Or did I ever even know how? Making my lunch is like lifting concrete. Walks never refresh me (they used to, didn't they?). Food turns to dust in my mouth. I try talking to my coworkers, but I feel drunk, or like I'm talking through a wall, or a pool of molasses. It's exhausting to form a sentence and, when I'm finished it, I'm out of breath. Do they notice? Am I talking slowly? More quietly? Do I look as delusional as I feel? What's wrong with me? I think something's wrong with me.

I don't work. I sit and stare, unable to move, unable to make any decisions, consumed by my thoughts. I look at the people around me, tirelessly typing away on their computers, taking calls late into the night like what they're doing actually matters.

We're all just slowly killing ourselves, I think. We all just work jobs we hate, longing for weekends until we die. Everyone I love is either going to move away from me or die. Everything I love is going to end, and the end is real and unbearably close.

I go home, having accomplished nothing, desperate to feel some relief, some familiarity. There's nothing. I'm alone, which crushes me. I lie on the floor on the front mat and can't move, no matter how much I berate myself. I go to bed. I hope I don't wake up tomorrow.

I read books, articles, blog posts, trying to unstuck myself. Okay. Be kind to yourself. One day at a time. Find something to look forward to. But there's nothing. Everything is a stale cracker—food, music, reading, writing, friends—all stale crackers. I enjoy nothing. I've lost everything, including myself. If I can't do the things that make me me, who am I? Texts come in, asking me how I'm doing, what I've been writing, reading, doing. Each one is a stab of accusation. Look at you, they accuse, look at all the things you're not doing. You're even failing at being yourself.

I go on medical leave from work. I move back with my family. I'm the ultimate failure; I can't handle a grown-up job or grown-up living on my own, and I never will again. I've ruined my life, and there's no recovery. Everything is my fault. I'll never get another job or be happy again. I hate myself for acting like a child and feel guilty that I feel so awful when there are so many others experiencing so much worse. I don't deserve to allow myself to feel like this. I resent that I can't take care of myself. No one understands, no one can ever understand. I'm alone and will always be alone.

I. Am. Alone.

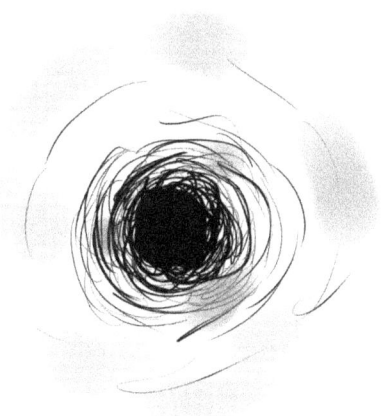

A selfish, hateful monster has overtaken my brain and crowded out every other thought. I curl into myself, further and further, in an attempt to not let the monster spill out and attack the people around me. It comes out anyway, gnashing its teeth, screaming and crying and scratching.

I want to run away, but mostly from myself. I repeat *escape* in my head. Sleep is a temporary relief, so I do that often, but it's not enough. The only way out is death—could the river wash me away? What if I stepped off the curb a moment too soon? Anything could be better than this hell-filled hopelessness. I lose myself in the internet and the lives of other people, hating myself and hating them for their lives, living while I'm not. I wish desperately to go back, for this to end, for things to be different. A dark black haze buzzes in my brain and my eyes, pushing out all other thoughts so I can't concentrate on anything else, can't remember anything else. The world was always this black. I know the truth now. I sink deeper and deeper.

Finally, I stop.

I wake up slowly. I wake after being tended to, held and patiently loved and waited for. There's no out. Life is here, and there are people here, for now. They drop off letters that I read and don't reply to. They send cards and texts. They don't ask too many questions, but they're there. I take steps—like pulling teeth. I make a list of things I don't want to do (I've always been good at lists), and do them, one by one. Calling doctors, sitting in the shame and embarrassment of failure, guilt, procrastination, hate, and crazy. I'm lucky that my people listen—doctors, family, friends.

I go for walks with my sister. I hide my hateful thoughts. I accept where I am, as messy as it is, and stop wishing to go back. I stop wishing for escape. I recognize things might not get better, but I will try, because I don't know if they will or not.

I try another medication—because what else is there to do—even though I know it won't work, because nothing does. I talk. I pick up the meds a month late. I walk. I start to wake up; the meds work. The sky looks blue, real blue again, not like I forgot to wake up and am half living in a dream. I start to feel excitement again, and I roll it around on my tongue, feeling its freshness like a freshly picked strawberry, something I never thought I'd experience again. I roll through each small happiness with burning gratefulness. I'm still alive and once again thankful to be.

A text comes through: *We're proud of you for getting through this.* Proud of me? For what? What did I do? I did nothing for months, stagnant and hating myself while the world moved on without me.

They didn't though. They were there, the whole time, waiting and loving and hoping. Who are you when you can't do anything, when you can't do the things that make you you: cooking and reading and being there for your friends and family and organizing things and giving and sharing and laughing?

You. Are. Loved.

And it means more in those moments, when I'm ugly and angry and can't give anything and don't deserve it. It is a godly, sacred kind of love.

Now awake, I can recognize the lies my brain piled on me. It comes in two words: *of course*. *Of course*, I want to live. *Of course*, there are many, many people who have been here before. *Of course* there are people who understand. *Of course* I'm capable, and I won't feel like this forever. *Of course*, I'll read, and write, and feel myself again.

And I am absolutely, definitively, not alone.

depression translations

this isn't like you

i know you can do these things

you need to figure out what you need

everyone's struggling

but you're so young

you have your whole life ahead of you

it's just like a broken leg
an easy fix

it gets better

it's okay to not be okay

please don't do anything stupid

you're not thinking straight

you've just had a nervous breakdown

it's okay to do nothing

there's a light at the end of the tunnel

we love you

i don't know where she went

pretty sure i killed her

you're alone and no one will help you

you're nothing special
      you're nothing

you're an immature child

        and you know nothing

it's not a big deal
    just put a cast on and get over it

well it's mostly gotten worse so far
        so i guess that's just not for me then

i am a failure and i did this to myself

you're weak and ignorant

great
    i'm failing at doing something
          as basic as thinking

you're a fucking wimp

i am useless and have no value

i guess i'm just uselessly blind then

i know i know i know

fix

i got hooked on a solution once
it fed me, elated me
i was a god
riding high on firm feet planted
there was nothing i couldn't figure out

one solution didn't satisfy
now i scour the internet for answers
hoard advice and methods and therapies
intoxicated on erasing questions
one by one by one by one

every depressed person i can make happy
every problem i can solve
i am the god of equations
meditation + exercise = i'm done now
i'm here i made it i've arrived

nothing's working anymore
i swallow all the complicated colours
i black out for awhile
when i wake up the world is black and white
and i can measure the world with certainty

why does this grey still exist
i thought i'd consumed it
i shake without explanations
i pace inhaling the why how what when
puff after puff after puff with no end

chest constricting, mouth dry, heart squeezes
crawling crazed, desperate scrambling
sick and shaking and sheet white
searching for anything
answer, switch, a magic wand

i found it i found it
the perfect answer
the end of it all
this will solve everything
the ultimate soluti—

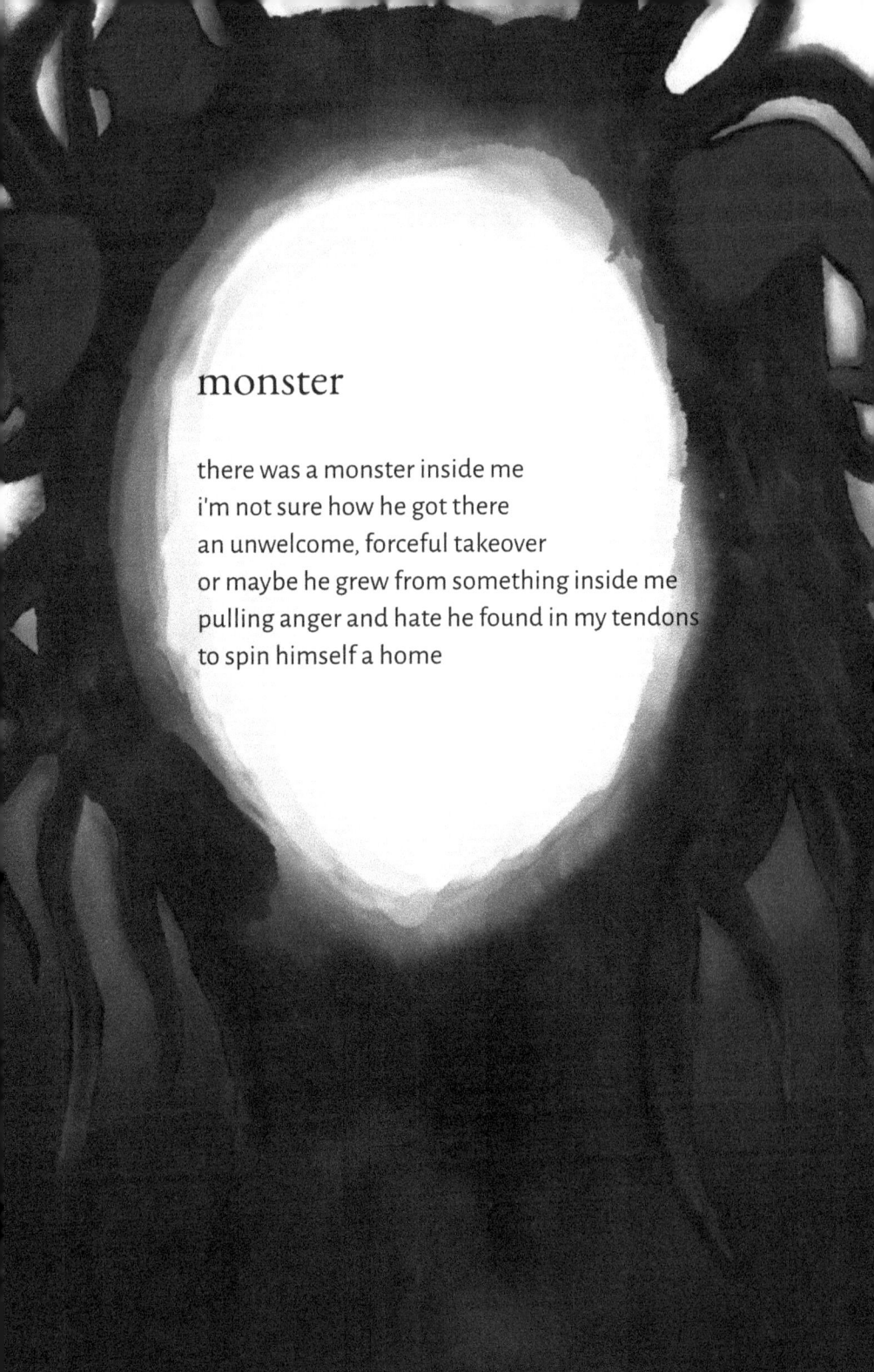

monster

there was a monster inside me
i'm not sure how he got there
an unwelcome, forceful takeover
or maybe he grew from something inside me
pulling anger and hate he found in my tendons
to spin himself a home

he strung me up, dragged me to destruction
pulled me to edges and screamed at me to leap
he raked my flesh with his long sharp talons
agonizingly tore open my flesh organs, muscles
becoming raw open wounds

he told me i will only let you go if you leave them
you hate them, he said (i *hate* them)
no i love them i want to stay
but he was drowning me with poison
hateful toxins filling me to my neck to choke me

i think he's gone now but i'm not sure
wasn't it i who let him in?

maybe he was always a part of me
maybe i'm just kidding myself
maybe he's just me

recovery

i crawl slowly from the endlessness of the dark, sickly caves and finally find myself blinking in the light. here, i'm a hollow eggshell, braced for a gentle tap that will shatter me into chipped pieces. i can see the light now, but will it last? is this careful stepping a sign? i'm a set bomb, and if impacted i'll explode, shooting out shrapnel to shred everything around me. i hold the light nervously, afraid that if i grip it too tightly, it'll burst.

you held my hope

you held my hope
in the meticulous watering of plants
in gentle nurturing
in patient waiting
for the eventual birth of green gifts

you held my hope
tight against kicks and screams and sobs
in your strong arms
in your warm touch
which soothes my angry red skin

you held my hope
folded in thirds and tucked in an envelope
written on a piece of lined loose-leaf
you dropped it in the mailbox
waited for me to pick it up

you held my hope
in the virtual space of dropped connection
in the tether you unravelled
dangling comforting threads
knotted to plump emoji hearts

you held my hope
in the love you held in your heart

you held my hope until
i could find it again

and because you held my hope

i found it

not far

these little things

walking, boots crunching dead leaves, trading life stories

using a new umbrella

the crackle of a fire, hair absorbing bonfire smoke

rubbing fluffy cat bellies, burying my face in fur

mornings spent basking in sunshine and writing, tea in hand

clean sheets

plants that grow with little encouragement

friends dropping off melt-in-your-mouth cookies in yogurt containers

a good sleep

when someone comes home and you get to talk about your day

learning something new about someone

reading a good book in one sitting

when the house smells like sweet cinnamon and sugar

thunderstorms

a freezer full of on-sale ice cream bars

sitting at a desk that looks out a window

walking to work and enjoying the fresh air

spotting a woodpecker in the trees

avocados

a note on the fridge that says "help yourself to brownies"

waking up and not having to be anywhere

doing morning yoga with my sister

a package on the step with my name on it

a new book i've been waiting to read for ages

well-narrated audiobooks

a good, filling dinner with farm-fresh vegetables

a perfectly blended smoothie

a TV show that makes me laugh and love and cry and want to make art

biking down the street on a cool day realizing i'm propelling myself
     with my own bodily strength

fairy lights in the porch at night

dinner's ready when i get home from work, starving

rest

shatter the chains of striving
break open filled time
and the constant clinging to becoming more by doing
which pulls your skin taut against your bones

disentangle yourself from twisted truths
recklessly release and relieved, enter into this
a fierce and powerful
resistance

impaction (life jumping)
Erin Toews

Perched on the edge of a cliff,
I hesitate, gauging the distance
from where I am to where I'll jump.
The water below is unclear,
an impenetrable brown-grey;
who knows if I'll be crushed
against a hidden rock,
or if the lake is shallow?

I know that billions have leapt before
and made it alright.
I know that my faith could be quenched at the bottom.
But some, a few, tipped in the air,
collapsed and impacted,
resurfaced half-conscious and sodden.

See, my legs can't make me leap
because my heart stops them,
and my head;
they've been stilled and smalled
to evade the jump,
so I remain stuck,
self-conscious and beheld.

If this cliff was a catalyst,
I would understand my fear,
but it's only a small rock,
one of many that I look over
and leap off every day.

the process of self-love

i am drawn in window fog
impermanent, feckless figure,
transparent and temporary,
evaporates by midday

a frisson in the veins
skin, clothes, accepted script
conceals the inner soul;
safer if kept sequestered

the world a judge
only there to conspire
against those who attempt
a naive confidence

exposing truth to air
only causes rust, leaving
the stomach-twisting taste
of iron on the tongue

why unclothe layers of deceptive armour
when hiding is comfortable:
room enough to breathe,
preferable to rejection

beneath
the pith of self remains—
unexplored

restoration
Erin Toews

> "...'My grace is sufficient for you, for my power is made perfect in weakness'..."
> —2 Corinthians 12:9 (NIV)

My heart is like a jar of clay
but shattered, now in shards
that launched like shrapnel through my chest
and cut me to the ground.

In between great gasps of pain,
I see the Potter waiting,
holding his tool for mending high,
an offering.
I resist—"No need. I'm fine."—
but the pain continues on and on
and so I beg him, "Come."

Gingerly, he picks out the pieces,
tenderly, he glues them with gold.
"This will hold," he says
and lays my heart in me.
In awe, I touch my broken heart
now whole, revealing veins—restored.

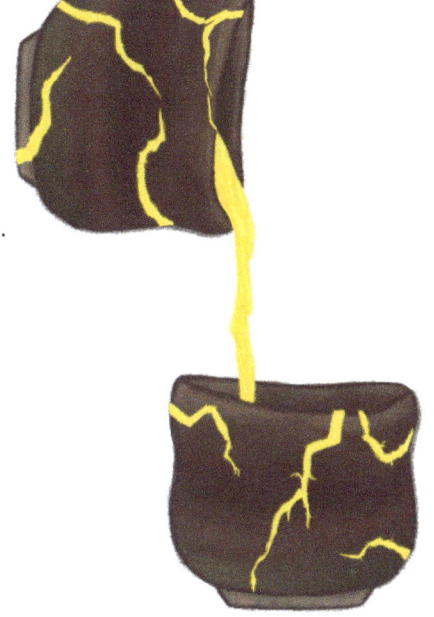

twins: 15 months apart
Amelia Warkentin

So similar, you my mirror.
We talk and we laugh.
We both name our fears.

We've both had our struggles.
Both wrestled with pride,
both fought inner demons-unseen-inside.

When we rage war with our own minds,
we'll care for others, but to ourselves, we're unkind.

(You haven't been yourself lately, I fear I know what this means.
Sometimes your past battles still haunt my dreams.)

When mental illness first took you,
your eyes were empty and wide,
now they portray the pain you wrestle inside.

That first time I held you, hummed hymns in your ears.
Now we talk briefly—in phone calls—through tears.

That first time I was jealous, was sick—selfish too,
Now I wish there was more I could do,
to free you from yourself.

twins: 15 months apart
Amelia Warkentin

So similar, you my mirror.
We talk and we laugh.
We both name our fears.

We've both had our struggles.
Both wrestled with pride,
both fought inner demons-unseen-inside.

When we rage war with our own minds,
we'll care for others, but to ourselves, we're unkind.

(You haven't been yourself lately, I fear I know what this means.
Sometimes your past battles still haunt my dreams.)

When mental illness first took you,
your eyes were empty and wide,
now they portray the pain you wrestle inside.

That first time I held you, hummed hymns in your ears.
Now we talk briefly—in phone calls—through tears.

That first time I was jealous, was sick—selfish too,
Now I wish there was more I could do,
to free you from yourself.

how to measure friendship

by distance?
the number of footsteps to a neighbour's door
no farther than an arm's reach
or a leg stretching to kick a snoring roommate
person plus proximity?

by time?
here with you from waking to sleeping
missing a minute means our unmooring
the longer we stand together
the more melded our hearts?

by knowledge?
textbooks of answers to mundane questions
your favourite colour is blue since when
how many blanks I can fill on your forms
the number of memorized facts?

by interactions?
hey, smile, name, nod
basic acknowledgement of existence
brief connections eventually counted
as something more?

by depth?
meters descended into your soul
heart laid bare enough to see all your scars
how far i've fallen
into the agony of your existence?

by silence?
diving deep into a chasm of no words
trying to find telepathic understanding
how many ounces of courage
and not giving up?

please give me
a ruler a scale a beaker
container to capture
make me sure of what i have
to the decimal place

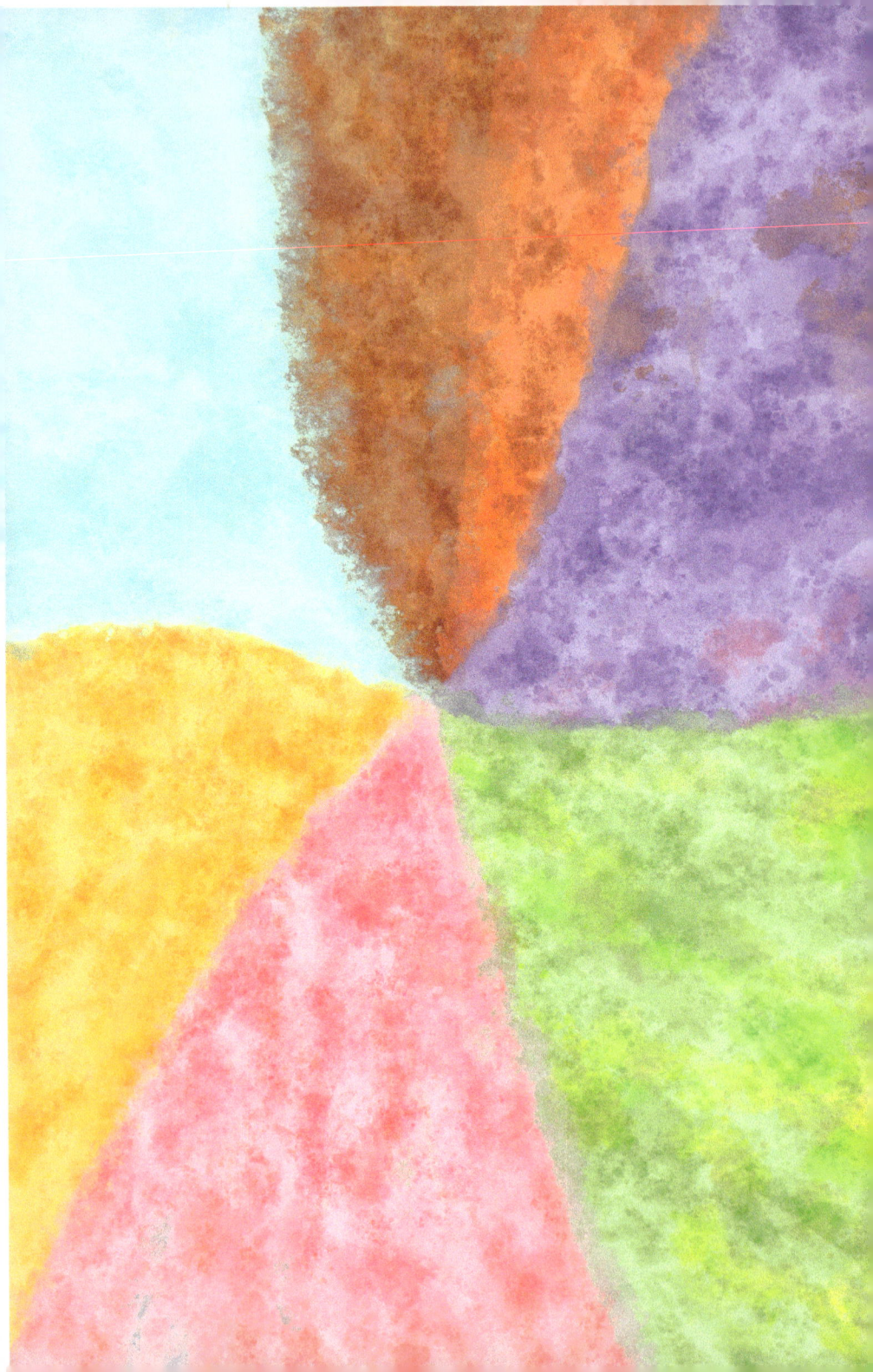

Chicago (with you)

city fades
skyscrapers recede from the skyline
music decrescendos into the distance
until there's just
you
reminding me of how i wished and got
more than i could ask or imagine

you
reminding me what hope looks like

the faith of the matriarch

My grandmother Dorothy inspired a lot of my life, and one of the things that I always admired about her was her quiet, gentle faith, which she lived out through loving and connecting with others, and through committed friendship. Growing up in an Evangelical church, I found that the most admired Christians were the ones who had the highest conversion tally. But, through my grandmother, I experienced another way of living out my faith. Gentleness and kindness are not often associated with power in today's world, but that was my grandmother. And she was the most powerful person I knew. She could make anyone do anything, and she could connect with anyone.

I remember sitting in her apartment living room when I was younger, sipping orange pekoe tea while she told me stories of when she and Grandpa lived in Australia when they were first married. She told me a story about meeting a young Chinese woman on the boat to Australia, and how that woman and her husband became good friends with them. I asked what happened to that couple, and was awestruck to learn that Grandma still kept in touch through letters and phone calls. Their friendship wasn't a distant memory at all, like I had assumed it would be. Because of her example, I've committed myself to keeping up with my friends in the same way.

When I was younger, I would go to Round Lake with my grandparents and some of my dad's extended family. We would travel five hours into the rolling hills of Saskatchewan to spend weekends, or sometimes weeks, at a rustic cottage on the beach. My family and the family of our Auntie Corinne would squish into the tiny, two-bedroom cabin and while away the weekend playing games and exploring the outdoors.

I would spend most of my time with my cousin, Auntie Corinne's granddaughter. We would come up with creative ideas while the adults napped, one of which involved my cousin dressing up in a sheet and putting on a play I wrote called "The Nightingale." Sometimes, I would try to connect in my head how exactly I was related to my cousin, trying to put together a seemingly nonsensical family tree.

As it turned out, I couldn't figure it out, because my "cousin's" family were not actually related to us by blood. Auntie Corinne was my grandmother's long-time friend, from the time they were 10 years old. Somehow, even though they were disconnected by provincial borders, they, and eventually their respective families, stayed intertwined. My dad and his siblings spent endless summers as kids at the lake with Auntie Corinne and her sons, and once they all had kids, we spent time there too. Eventually, summers at the lake dwindled to nothing as the cabin was repeatedly battered by flooding, but the two matriarchs kept their families connected through occasional trips for celebrations or hockey games, or grand once-every-four-years weekend Thanksgivings. Auntie Corinne and Grandma were as close as sisters.

At Auntie Corinne's funeral, her son reached across and laid a hand on my dad's arm and said, "Don't worry, you're blood," and led us into the back of the church where the rest of the family were gathering. My grandmother and Auntie Corinne's incredibly strong bond of friendship lived on for 90 years.

In the last two years of her life, my grandma had a stroke that left her paralyzed, using a wheelchair, and living in a personal care home with my grandpa, who was also losing his capabilities. Her slightly damaged memory and body didn't stop her, although her personality was a bit different and the filter that made her present herself as proper had been stripped away by brain damage.

Despite her new disabilities, my grandma became the darling of her personal care home, to no one's surprise. She knew everyone, staff or resident, and everyone knew her. She would wheel down the hall on her floor, softly saying names and brushing fingertips of those not quite present like some kind of saint. She had a gift for making people feel comfortable sharing their lives and their struggles with her. In turn, she shared with them her faith and confidence in God, mostly through actively showing God's compassion to those around her.

My dad told a story at her funeral about when she had a seizure and ended up in the hospital, something that happens sometimes after a stroke. By 1:30 in the morning, my dad was the only one left with Grandma, and she continued talking even as late as it was. A nurse came to wheel Grandma away for another test. After 15 minutes, they returned to the room my dad was waiting in. Grandma was chatting with the nurse as an old friend, saying how she was sure she would do well in her courses, and she would definitely get the job she wanted, and that she hoped her son would continue to improve. The woman thanked her, said "Take care, Dorothy," and left.

My dad asked where Grandma knew the nurse from. Grandma replied that actually they had only just met, right now, and had talked in the 15 minutes as they walked to and from the test. My dad marvelled at how Grandma, in the time most people would only have barely got past the weather, had connected with the nurse in a way that allowed her to be comfortable sharing her dreams and fears.

But that was just Grandma—open and honest and gentle and gracious and so, so strong to be able to connect on that level with everyone she met: family, friends, and strangers who were really just future friends.

Subconsciously and consciously, I have modelled my life after my grandmother's and the way she connected with others. All the cards or letters I've sent to friends over the years in an effort to keep in touch and remind them of my love for them are because of her. Any meal I've hosted to bring people together, where I attempt (and usually fail) to perfect the presentation is because of her. Any friendship I've worked to maintain for years, despite hardship, has been because of her. Every decision I've made not to give up on someone has been because of her gracious, kind, and compassionate example.

If I can accomplish anything in my life, I hope to leave as strong a legacy of faith shown through love as my grandmother did, even if it might look a little bit different.

dear grandma

did you know
when you and she were schoolmates
neighbours playing on the front step
making mud pies
how much everything would change

did you know
that you would both fall in love
follow your men to far-off places
write letters to close the distance
between the dark and unknown ocean

did you know
that you would make a new home in a strange land
that time would make her a stranger to your first child
she'd meet him five years later
you undecided if this meeting is already too late

did you know
that the separation wouldn't last
that you'd spend hours together in a cabin
your kids intermingling
into one giant messy family

did you know
that you would do everything together
wear matching multicoloured muumuus
walk side-by-side to the two-hole cabin outhouse
play endless hours of Scrabble which she always won

did you know
that the red-trimmed cabin would crumble
battered by age and high tides
time lapping the edges
pulling you both apart

did you know
your bodies would betray you
you'd lose your freedom to locked doors
that you would speak too quietly into the phone
and she couldn't hear you anymore

did you know
that after 90 years of friendship
you'd die three months apart
both having stood after your husbands departed
your souls still threaded, tugging after each other

did you both know
when you and her were schoolmates
neighbours playing on the front step
making mud pies
how you and her would change everything

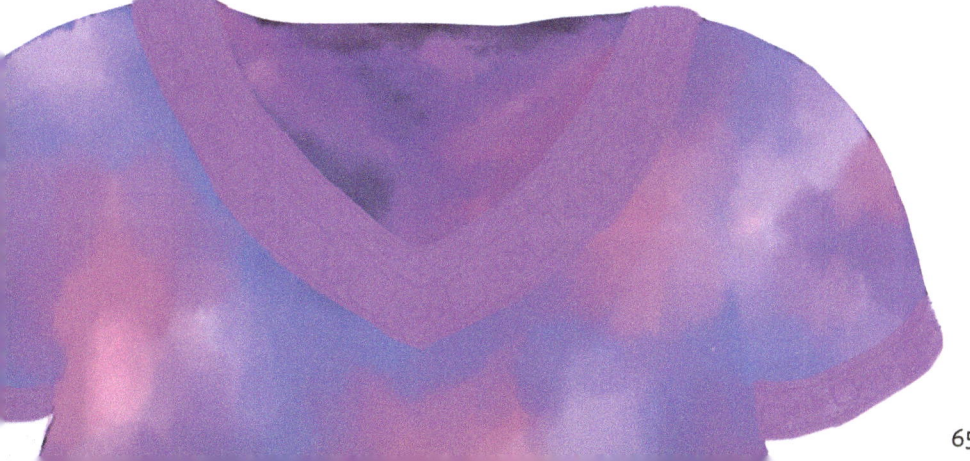

heartbreak

I've never been good at letting go. I always assume every friend I make will be my friend forever and that transient relationships are the result of not trying hard enough. People say that friends can grow apart, but I never want to believe them. Because of my grandmother and my parents' fierce admonishments that my siblings and I hold our commitments seriously, I never, ever want to give up on anyone. I want to believe that I can make things stay the same forever, because with change comes the terrifying unknown. But inevitably, things change. When I graduated high school, I was terrified of losing my people. I did end up losing a few, and it hurt like hell.

The first was a friend of mine with whom I had grown up in church. We had spent years giggling in church pews about youth group crushes and emailing back and forth about everything and nothing, all the while marvelling at the very, very different backgrounds we came from. We appreciated each other nonetheless.

When she told me that her boyfriend, soon-to-be fiancé, was her best friend, it shattered me. I was supposed to be her best friend. How could that happen? We had been soulmates for years, since we were seven or eight years old, and now this stranger was replacing me? I covered my hurt and jealousy with anger at her giving into her weakness for boys and abandoning me. Didn't she know that she didn't need a man to complete her?

I didn't understand her desire for a relationship at the time, and likely she didn't understand my complete disinterest in one. I loved my friends and didn't need a partner. I've come to realize that pursuing relationships isn't a failure of independent womanhood, but merely another life decision, another path you can take that can be just as messy as any other. It's just unfortunate that partnership and marriage are much more often represented in media instead of lasting friendship. Movies often end after the couple gets together, because the end goal of life is presented as partnership. We've structured our society around marriage, and church groups are often split between single people and married couples.

Perhaps I find it so hard to let go because my friendships are the main relationships that sustain me, rather than a partner or a spouse. I would love for my connections with others to be more recognized in society. My friendships may be just as intense and committed as any marriage, yet I don't get multiple parties, or legal documents, or the recognition or concreteness of a ceremonial commitment. Instead, I have to accept the weird fluctuations, uncertainty, and loneliness of being single, something I don't resent precisely because of the love that surrounds me. Still, the heartbreak of losing a friendship to partnership is very, very real.

It took me a long time to come to terms with the grief of change in friendship—mourning a past dynamic while being nervous and uncertain of the new one. My old friend and I are actually still friends today. Since she has three kids now, we see each other once every six months or so, and we talk about our families and update each other on our lives while kids interrupt us every five minutes. We are different, and acknowledge the different paths we have taken in our lives; her pursuing motherhood and church ministry as a pastor's wife, and me pursuing university education and career. I spent a long time hurt and grieving the change in our friendship, but now I have come to accept that it will not be like it was before, but can still be okay in the future, if different. I've also come to accept that I can't hold onto everyone. I'm only human, and my hands are only so big. I have to let go and trust that the love I gave they still, in some way, carry with them.

forgive

gut reaction: revolt
harbour hurts as a handful of arrows
pile them up for protection
except you're the one being pierced

upon reflection: bury all weapons
debris from collapsed story endings
leave behind graves of what ~~could have been~~ never was
believe in beginnings

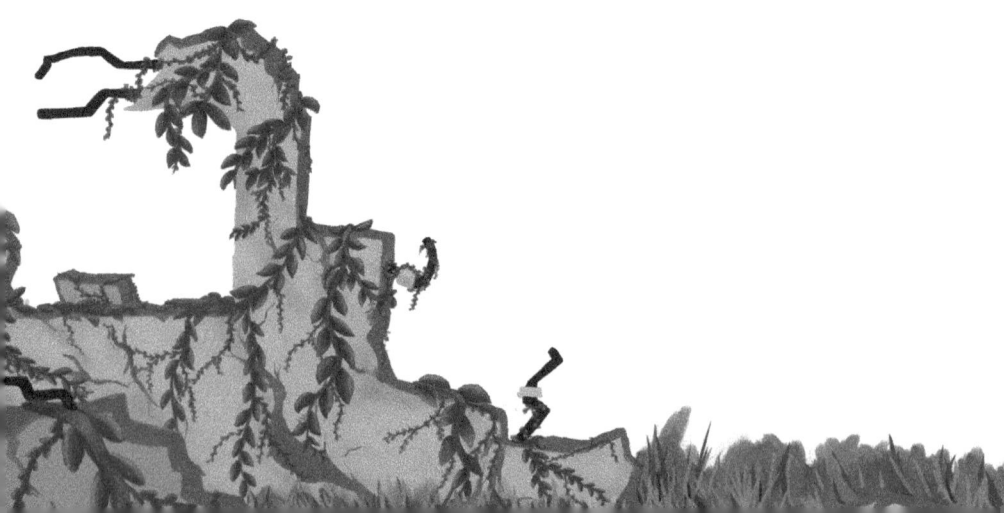

grown up

suddenly i blink
five years have passed
and you've changed
i thought i'd been keeping track
and i'd still be able to recognize you

we are like the blobs
in a lava lamp
pulling apart
and coming together
making different shapes each time

waves

We begin as capillaries, gentle ripples in a tide pool, a drop of vast ocean. We encircle and find each other, two of us linking up, then three, then five, then seven, until we are a group. We connect in our shared nerdiness, misfit identities, and disregard of middle school popularity politics. For now, we are classmates, lunch time buddies. We are unaware of how we might settle into each other. For now, we are young, we play, and it all comes easy.

The tide pool grows a little bit, and so do we, inching ever closer to the grand ocean and all its mysteries that await us. There are other things that occupy our time, but it's easy to stay together when we're locked in the same building day after day. We operate on a similar script, one we all know. We can complain about the same teachers, gossip about the same fellow students, and gather in the same cafeteria or library during breaks from class. We all know the language of this world.

The tide comes in, and we all roll slowly out to sea. This is the time when people disappear on their journeys, tumbling to many different shores. We break apart, some of us wandering far and others temporarily making place in warmer waters. We sustain ourselves through long, rambling emails and refuse to forget each other. There's always the question—will the sea be too large, too wide, too strong? Will we be able to survive its brutal battering, its unpredictable storms?

We are the waves, roiling in and out, swirling around each other. Sometimes one of us drifts out for a while, but they eventually return to kiss the sand. We crash into each other, then break apart. Our waters all mix in different ways, curling currents coming and going. We go different ways, pursuing different studies or careers, settling into our unique yet similar convictions and each trying to find meaning where we can. The similar school script has long been obliterated, and sometimes we have to find a new language. Often, we rely on a melancholy nostalgia, trying to recreate the time when everything was familiar even though we didn't necessarily know ourselves. The sad echoes of what once was fall flat.

We integrate more into the saltwater, becoming the strength of the ocean, plunging, surging, collapsing, feeling its difficulties, the way it consumes life, but also finding new people within. We're all a part of different worlds now, and we crash down on the environments we find ourselves in, trying with incomparably minuscule slaps to move a few mountains. We alternate lifting each other up, carrying hurts and victories, and sharing pride in the ways we find each other shifting the world.

It's been over 15 years and we still somehow find ourselves swirling around each other, moving in and out like the tide but always, somehow, together. When we were eddies in the tide pool, we may not have picked each other to spend the next 15 years with. How did this happen? A shared value, the fact that we stayed in the same geographical space, shared lasting singleness, just the fact that we had people willing to work at basic logistics? Some strange magic?

The ocean stretches out before us, black and deep and fathomless. With faith, we will continue to swirl around each other. But, for now, we don't delve too deep into mysteries. We dream of our 80-year-old selves, knitted blankets on our laps, still laughing and sharing and knowing. For all we know that will stay a dream. The ocean lives on, though, crashing and swirling, continuing to scoop up new young, naive ripples and tossing them out to sea.

kindred spirits

Manila, Philippines, 2012

We met in the parking lot. It was another humid, sunny tropical day, but your bright joy outshone it without effort, enrapturing me immediately. I had been waiting for you, hoping this student teacher from from Canada might be the one to fill the loneliness. This loneliness had filled me for the past three months while I volunteered at the international school and lived with my aunt and uncle in a small three-room on-campus apartment. Your smile was wide and held laughter and an endless, mesmerizing joy. You hugged me—we had just met, and yet you hugged me with all the enthusiasm and familiarity of a good friend—and from then on, we were. I already loved you.

Hundred Islands, Philippines, 2013

A year of shopping trips, afternoon coffee, Korean ice cream runs, late night Wizard games with friends, beach trips, friendships, Bible studies, and laughter. Two weeks of being roommates during which we whispered to each other about faith, and loneliness, and relationships at night. I told you I thought I could be happy being single for the rest of my life, and you didn't blink. I felt the coldness and emptiness in the room when you went back to your house and your roommate there. Here, a day of swimming, snorkelling and sunburn in some of the most beautiful locations in this country, with fresh delectable food to match. At night, we tucked into our shared bed—three women, two men and my aunt and uncle sharing one room at the resort to save money—and giggled under the covers about whether we'd wear our bras all night or not when there were *boys* in the room. Warm smiles and the wonder of how I could feel so utterly comfortable being myself with someone I'd known less than a year, even as it made perfect sense.

New Brunswick, Nova Scotia & Prince Edward Island, Canada, 2014

A year later, I visited you in your home and experienced your world. I got to watch you dance with abandon at a music festival, interact with your friends, listen to your beautiful singing in your church. The people at your church asked me why I was there—to see you, I said, and they seemed surprised. We harmonized while we watched the rolling Atlantic Ocean waves crash against the red rocks, we sludged illegally through mud flats with the Hopewell Rocks at our backs, and we walked through the Haunted Woods of Green Gables, two present-day kindred spirits re-imagining the close kinship of Anne and Diana from long ago.

Winnipeg and Moncton, Canada, 2014–2018

The harshness of being close every day for a week to separate lives again, with the uncertainty and unknown of the future—would we come back together again, ever? Occasional texts, the excitement of a letter or a card in the mail, and the frustration of lagging Skype connection. All I wanted was you in the present, so I didn't miss any words and I could hug you. The time and distance was long and hurt, but the love was strong enough even as we continued to grow away from each other.

Chicago, United States, 2018

We'd been sustained by texts and occasional Skype calls for four years—would it be enough? Would it be the same? But we immediately fell into the same trust and comfort that first brought us together. We talked about faith and God and trust. We lay on the grass in Millennium Park, almost getting our heads stepped on, *My Fair Lady* playing on stage while we talked about optimism and hope for the future. I aspired after your hopefulness. We sat next to the fountain and took silly selfies, we walked and walked and sometimes snipped at each other but ultimately forgave.

Mostly, we got to do life together, something missing from growing up in parallel, provinces away. We ate and prayed and argued and got to make decisions together. I saw your headaches and silliness; you saw my judgmental and selfish side. We annoyed each other sometimes or often. I found out you like to walk fast and keep moving, and you clench your teeth in your sleep. We sang together and talked about dumb mundane things that made up the everyday that we missed with each other for years.

On the plane ride home, I felt the goodbye as a physical ache. How could everyone on the plane be so normal when I was being crushed by the heartbreak of separation from my kindred spirit? I wanted to shout, cry, but instead I looked out the plane window at the city disappearing through the cloud below and held the ache as a gift.

Ottawa, Canada, 2020

This week is a restful settling in the midst of our busy lives. We recognize that we will continue to grow and change, but we will always in some ways grow together. Like an old married couple, we nestle into long-term comfort while always exploring new discoveries. We spend hours walking, and hours on the couch watching episode after episode of *Community*. I have no doubt now that we'll last, whatever that may look like or wherever we may go. I'm proud of you. I admire you, and hope for you, and love you.

My kindred spirit.

tilt-a-whirl
Erin Toews

Drugs? Please.
Caffeine and my best friends—
these I'll always take
to help induce euphoria.

The feeling's similar
to spinning in a cup,
clutching at its rim,
pushed and left to whim
of centrifuge and pulled
in by centripetal
force, opening
your eyes to see the earth
a looping go-kart course,
whooping, slightly sick,
in desperate need of wits,
but not enough to stop
this feeling that you're twirling open
into bliss.

what really happened in Vancouver

I'm not very good at telling people about my travel adventures. Or maybe you just can't accurately tell people about the intense, stretching experiences you have when you leave home, explore new places, and get to know someone's heart. "Oh, yeah, how was your trip!" "Oh, so much fun!" But always so much more.

Have you ever had the experience of meeting someone and connecting with them within a couple of hours? You start out hesitant, unsure that you should have even said yes to this arranged meeting, but you immediately feel a strange sense of calm and comfortability in their joyfulness. Gently, you just talk, slowly allowing yourself to be peeled away until you reveal a small piece of your heart. And there you find a connection, that you both share a faith, that your values overlap, that you surprisingly want to spill more of your soul. You suddenly realize this person is lovely and joyous, and you're only supposed to have this one night, but you want more.

After that night, they go back home, three provinces over. You don't see them, but you keep in touch. Then, nine months later, you decide to go stay with them for a week. As you're packing to leave, you have a moment of panic, and momentarily think, *What have I done? I've gone and booked a trip to stay with a stranger for a week.* But then you remember that you liked this person, and you get excited all over again to explore these new shores, of the country and of your relationship.

I sound like I'm talking about falling in love with someone, which I guess is what it is. The way I do friendship is often a lot like falling in love: intense and overwhelming and emotional.

Getting to know someone you've connected with so well on a deep, heart level is strange. You feel like you've known them for years, and they know exactly how to analyze you, but they don't know basic things, like what colours you wear (they figure it out fast) or that you get motion sick—little things that all your friends already know about you.

It's a strange but beautiful experience. Vancouver's places in my mind are now linked with conversations that let me see into your heart, and everything exposed just made me love you more. We sat on a log beside the Museum of Anthropology at the University of British Columbia, looking out over a pond, a totem pole towering over us, keeping watch with the purple mountains in the distance, and we talked about mental health and eating disorders. I felt embarrassed over teasing you about your eating habits, and tried to fumble my way back, humbling myself to listen like I've had to do way too many times, and will have to do many more.

We drove through the windy, hilly back country roads of Victoria, watching the browned February branches and moss-covered trees whiz by, discussing culture and family and media and everything wrong with Hollywood. We rode on a basically empty bus at 7:30 in the morning, talking about idealism and realism and changing the world. We sat on the carpeted floor in a busy community centre, relaxing and teasing each other and discussing, opening up our worldviews and our history to each other, challenging each other, strengthening our bond with each sentence spilled. We sat on a bench in front of Canada Place, me in awe of the mountains, you not even noticing the magic. You laughed when I asked you, "How are you not intimidated by the mountains all the time?" because I felt their presence like a physical, inimitable force in the pit of my stomach.

We talked of our futures, of weddings and husbands and our views on relationships. On a sunny day, we sat in front of the water, I don't even know where, talking about faith and God and church, seeing the irony when an eager man in a camouflage jacket walked up and handed us tract cards that asked us where we'd go if we died. When we stood on the train, gripping the yellow pole when it jerked, you told me why your sister said once that you were demonic, how you were in such a bad place in Grade 12 that you ran away. I imagined you slightly younger, anger in place of your current laughter and innocence, hair in all directions, sitting on a train like the one we were standing on with bags surrounding you, angry and hating yourself, feeling alone. You said they found you in a Chapters of all places, looking up from a book you were reading to see your father and brother standing over you. I felt like someone had punched me in the gut; I resolved to pray for you.

We walked across the UBC campus at night, lugging our bags down an empty pathway lit along the way by lamps, a kids' sports team just emptying from one of the gyms of the university sports complex surrounding us. I made you laugh by being silly and free. I admitted I didn't think I had a dark side.

There are other moments, but because they are moments, they are many. I watched you and your mother bicker, amused but also wary. We worked separately on our computers in your apartment that smelled vaguely of Indian food and dead fish. You continuously said ridiculous things just to shock me because I had fallen for your sweet innocence. I watched as you somehow pulled smiles and laughter out of everyone that you passed on the street.

These things—the things that strengthen our heart ties, that somehow make us known to each other—these are the things I will remember from my trip to Vancouver the most. Not the amazing views, or the hiking, or the tours. I remember the person I did it all with.

long distance

friends stretching hearts across borders
a random text brushes fingertips through screens
mundane moments together
invisibly intertwined
life tiptoes on and maybe one day
you could be here

winter song

what if we holed up in a cottage somewhere
snowdrifts as high as the windows
inside we'd make snow pudding
like that one episode of Little Bear

loving you is less complicated than i thought
the soul searching has been done
all we need now
hot chocolate and trusted Frosty

served with love

I learned food as love from my grandparents and my communities. My maternal grandfather, Grandpa Friesen, was often missing from the thick hubbub of family gatherings as he was always glued in front of the stove or the barbecue, serious and straight-faced, taking control of whatever elaborate meal he was cooking up (usually a lot of meat). The kitchen was his no-nonsense domain and others would get reamed out if they overstepped. When I think of Grandpa now, the image in my mind is him with an apron adorning his stout, slightly pudgy frame, a barbecue flipper in one hand, asking shortly how everyone wants their steak done.

My grandpa was also notorious for offering more and more food, no matter how much you refused or how stuffed you said you were. Ice cream was his favourite dessert, and he piled serving bowls high with scoop upon scoop. "Just a little bit, thanks," was not a comprehensible phrase to him. It was such a big part of his life that ice cream, in tubs, was served at his funeral. Even in death he was filling people's stomachs to the brim.

My paternal grandmother, Grandma Sherlock, was known for her cooking and baking skills. They were legendary. Many of my family members have stories of making her recipes, only for them to not turn out right, even with her exact modifications. The magic of her food was impossible to reproduce. Exquisite roast, tender biscuits, perfectly-flavoured lemon blueberry muffins, with not so much of an ounce of blue juice bleed.

She was also a woman of presentation. No matter how something tasted, if it didn't look right, it went into the trash, much to the chagrin of the sweet-toothed men in her family. Her baking was impeccable; the reason I looked forward to Christmas every year was because of her dainties. I remember eating roasted vegetables of hers that were heavenly in their flavour and tenderness. I asked her how she did it, but didn't remember her instructions and never came to close to her excellence. I often wish I could still ask for her advice on how various cooking or baking techniques should work, or how to improve certain recipes. Or just to brag about my creations, feeble as they are in comparison to hers.

One of my favourite memories from the last two years of her life, after she had suffered her stroke, was putting together a lunch of egg salad, fruit, and homemade cookies and eating it together on the back patio of her personal care home on my birthday. I loved putting together something that I knew would make her happy. It was a way for me to give back a portion of what she gave me and many others over the years, a way to serve her the way she had served me.

When church members were sick, or had newborn babies, my church would put out a sign-up list for others to bring meals to them. My mom would double her dinner recipes only to pack half of it away in tinfoil for another family. Most of the cultures I've been surrounded by have an expectation of an overabundance of food. Scarcity of food is an affront, a sin, a horrible faux pas. Not bringing an embarrassment of riches to a potluck may come as close as Baptists will get to an excommunicable offence. Everyone must leave with their stomachs full enough that they can't walk properly, or the hosts or potluck contributors did their job wrong.

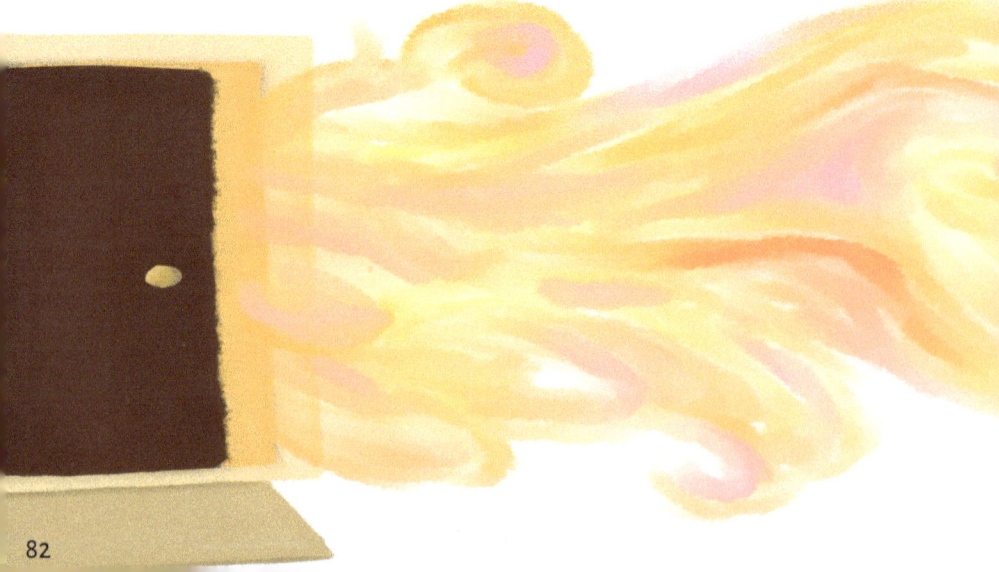

I experienced my first ever real, independent hosting in the Philippines. I had just spent a week over the school's October break with my aunt and uncle and three single school staff in Tagaytay, vacationing near a volcano. We played games and enjoyed the surprisingly cooler weather (we actually wore sweaters). When we got home, I noted that these women we had just spent the week with weren't often included in other "single staff" get-togethers. I desperately needed friends, so I asked my aunt if I could invite these three women, all a decade older than me, over for dinner. My mom gave me her taco casserole recipe (with the helpful tip of, "Well I don't really use a recipe though, and I make it differently every time"). My taco casserole turned out kind of watery, but it served its purpose. We gathered, we laughed, we played games—we began something that night. We became A Group. Those women became my best friends in the Philippines.

My aunt and uncle opened their home to all kinds of people. We had dinner guests multiple times a week, our table in our tiny three-room apartment packed with strangers becoming friends. I spent weeks at a time sharing my room with transient guests, getting to know people from all over the world. Through my aunt and uncle, I saw how offering hospitality could make people feel welcome and at home in a strange place. I was able to make close friends, far away from home after months of loneliness, by inviting a few strangers for dinner. Since then, I've loved to serve food to friends and host gatherings in an effort to continue the legacy of love that my grandparents began.

From these examples, I've always been cognizant of how food brings people together. Since I first learned how to cook, I've used food to give and serve love when I can't do anything else. If I can't fix, or take away, sadness or sickness, at the very least I can make food.

I value hospitality and love hosting, but I also know how I overcompensate with things out of my control. If I can do nothing else, I can feed people, make sure they are healthy, make sure they are okay. Making food provides me with a sense of worth and purpose, which is not always helpful when that accomplishment is not possible or welcome. Food, in that case, doesn't fix anything, but leaves me exhausted, especially when the best thing for me would be to just stop.

Maybe let someone feed me for a change, give others the opportunity to step up and care and show their strengths.

Regardless, when I invite you to my table, this is what it means:

I welcome you here. You are included in my heart and in my story. I give myself to you in this bread because I love you. You matter to me, so I'm going to do my part to sustain you. Here, you are served. Here, you are loved. Here, you are blessed. Please, come join me at my table and delight in this glorious feast.

desert girl in prairie summer storm
Erin Toews

For Amber, the desert-turned-prairie girl.

Raise your arms, desert girl,
dance in the rain.
Quickly as a pinwheel, twirl
and shriek into the sizzle.
Though this is only drizzle—
some drops of shock that douse
a strand of hair a minute, a blouse
within a half an hour—

soon it will pour, desert girl—
semi-opaque streaks
that crease the soil and overtake
the spotted circle pattern
stamped precisely by
the drizzle on the drive, and turn
biceps to rock beds for silken streams
and fingertips to waterfalls.
Echoes of lightning from distant
clouds will illumine your face
while rumbles of seconds-elsewhere thunder
buttress your joyous cries.

Embrace the rain, desert girl.
Rejoice, for here clouds
fall away and puddles dry,
yet always will return.

here's where i fell in love

In the stale windowless box of a cold workplace, I hide my insides, afraid to scare these new people away with my passions. Four days in, I stand in a circle of new co-workers and realize we're talking very seriously about Star Wars, and also, half the office plays D&D. I think I can maybe find a home here.

My grandma dies. The supposed leaders are cold, but everyone else is warm. The contrast shocks me to tears.

There's two of us alone in the office at the end of the day, and I hear a familiar, beloved podcast not from my speakers. "Are you watching Critical Role?" Forever after a connection.

Playful targeted insults, learning the office language of roasting and over-the-top sarcasm. Pranks and laughter, because sometimes you have to laugh when the only other option is to cry. After we finish the business part of our health and safety committee meeting, we spend time discussing a YouTube video of a cat licking a pickle. I write "improved office morale" in my daily activity log when we spend an hour and a half in the back office recommending fantasy books to each other.

Then, tumult and change and hurt and heartbreak and trying to hold on through splintering, consumed with worry that I won't have the strength. They all leave me. They need this; it's for the best. I'm in pieces.

A hand on an arm on the worst day and a sharing of tears and the creation of one of my favourite memories, ever. Things are different, my heart is numbed, but there are new friends. An unexpected connection with someone so different they seem slightly alien. Introducing a new, soft soul slowly, attempting to cushion her from the coldness.

Years later, I text with all of them every other day. I was so afraid, but I haven't lost them yet.

We sit around a table where the limits are only our imaginations. The leftover memories are of grand adventures, sweeping panoramas, vivid colours, dangerous battles, epic magic. The memories are incongruent with the photos of a bunch of nerds around a table cluttered with D&D mess and snacks. Somehow, the table is never big enough. In between romping fantasy adventures, we nap, restoring our bodies that have been zapped of energy from over-socialization. I keep talking, because I'm somehow the one in this group that can keep going, and because I'm happy. These sleepy moments in between are where we cuddle cats, and where the friendship fuses.

A global pandemic hits and everything stops. Suddenly, all we have is each other on screens on Friday nights. We escape blissfully into fantasy. My heart breaks that I only have to close my laptop on their faces to end the night. I feel a weird mix of longing and blessing when our characters hug in game. I want what they have, these imaginary people that exist in the liminal space of pretend.

I sit in a room with black walls that match the darkness that has leeched onto my brain and made it impossible for me to fully open my eyes. In our fantasy world, we're in a dark, corrupted forest, and we fight to the death. Explosions burst, and we are exhausted and broken to the bone. We take the enemy down, and we think we're safe, and then one final explosion goes off and one of us falls. There's nothing we can do. This is the end. In real life, in a nest of blankets on the floor, my face blue with screen glow, I realize that I cannot die, not yet.

I'm awake, and now we play in a world of cold ice. My character tries to push against the cold of everyone and everything around her with her warmth. Along adventures, she touches a cursed statue and becomes cursed herself. She becomes suspicious and paranoid of everyone around her. She is crazed and chaotic and not quite sure what's going on. I think, fleetingly, of how I acted only a few months before and notice the similarities.

My character snaps, driven to madness, possessed by darkness. Everyone around her brushes her off as crazy, sleep-deprived, drunk.

They don't listen to her foaming mad rants, but to her, it's oh so real. Eventually her friends take her to a doctor. The doctor listens, calms her down, gives her some herbs. The doctor is my friend, in real life, listening and giving me a gift, which my heart receives with tearful gratitude. I love my friends. I have experienced nothing like this moment, a piercing of reality into fantasy, a mingling of the two, and a beautiful, soulful miracle.

Under the high reaching arches of a musty church, I'm exhausted, not ready to put all my energy and concentration into a two-hour choir rehearsal, the weight of the week on my back. Chatter begins to bounce around the church sanctuary. Eventually, we gather in reflection and a moment of rest. This is the breath before the music begins, the moment in which I feel most strongly everything I've seen since I started with this misfit group of people two years ago. The acceptance without question, the confession of fears and difficulty without hesitation, the encouragement of pure, unhidden selves above all else. The fading away of masks from every other part of life. The love given, openly and comfortably.

Here, I become joyful, refreshed. I—we—sing love.

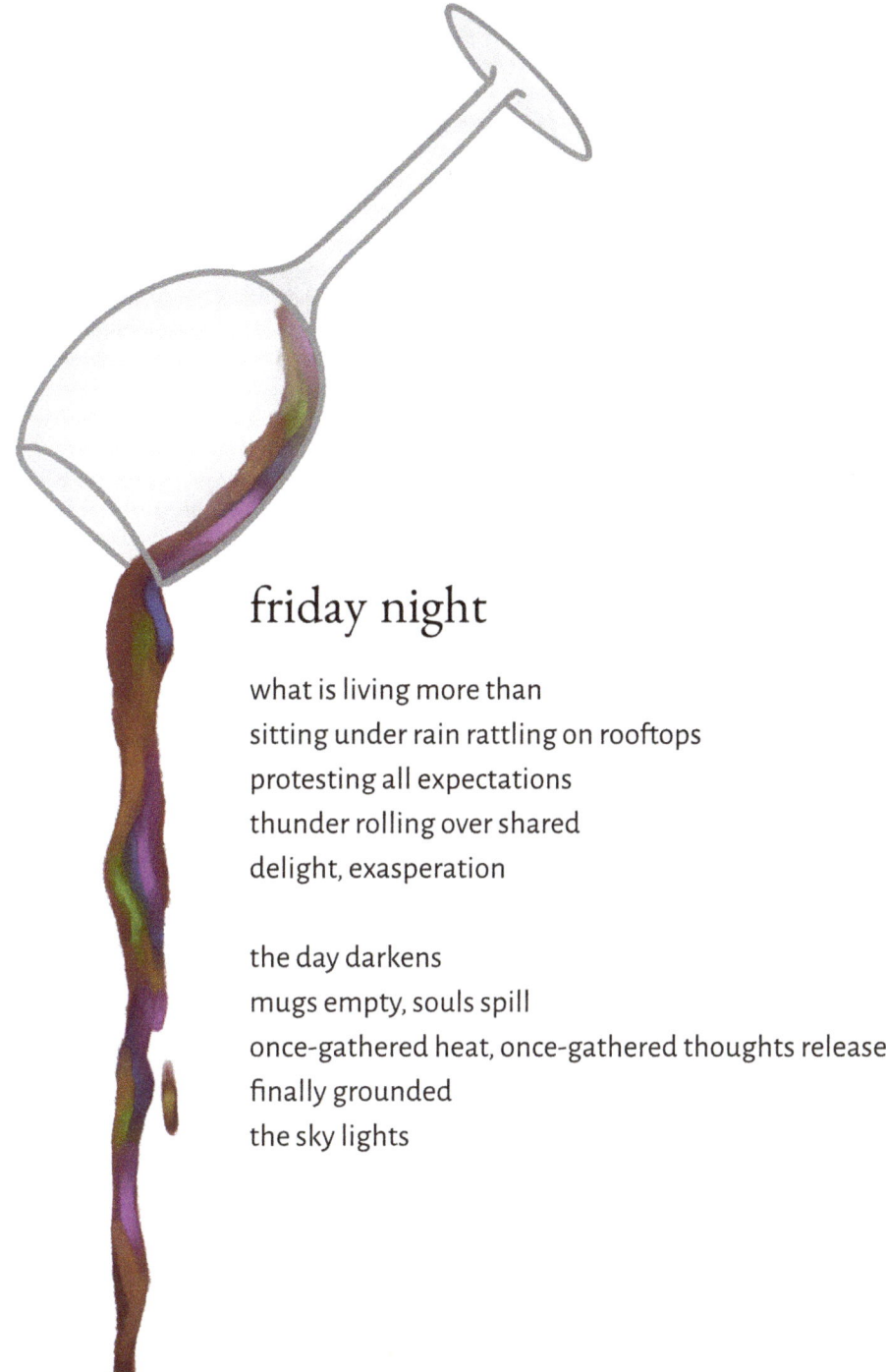

friday night

what is living more than
sitting under rain rattling on rooftops
protesting all expectations
thunder rolling over shared
delight, exasperation

the day darkens
mugs empty, souls spill
once-gathered heat, once-gathered thoughts release
finally grounded
the sky lights

resources that helped me

First of all, thank you to all of the people, friends, family, and internet personalities who have been open and honest about their mental health, illness, and recovery journeys. Talking about your experiences has helped me in ways I cannot express, even if it took a long time for me to be able to do the same. It makes me angry that there is still so much hidden away, by me and my own friends and family, as a result of the way the world is structured. Mental health and illness *needs* to be talked about. This book has been a step, for me, out into the open.

Getting professional help is by far the most difficult part of any mental illness recovery journey, but you can do it. If professional help is too overwhelming for you at the moment, please just tell someone you trust how you're feeling, and then talk to your doctor if you have that option. The first step is always the hardest. Everyone has mental health, and everyone should work to take care of it just as much as their physical health. I would also encourage you to look up what resources are available locally in your area. Please just start, and don't leave it as long as I did. If you have, it's not too late. These are some resources that helped me along my journey, and may be somewhere for you to start.

doddlevloggle, chattin' about therapy with tessa violet, https://www.youtube.com/watch?v=wmSon_pEqF8—This video helped me learn what therapy actually is, and it dispels a lot of therapy myths. I like how Tessa talks about thinking of therapy not in terms of, "Do I need it?" but "Do I want to better understand myself?"

Just Between Us, What OCD, Depression and Anxiety are Really Like, https://www.youtube.com/watch?v=qPY2mJV87NU—The open and honest way Gaby and Allison talk about mental illness and their experiences with recovery, such as medications and therapies, has been super helpful and eye-opening. They have a lot of videos on their channel about their first-hand experiences with OCD, depression, anxiety, and bipolar disorder.

Iz Harris, I Take Antidepressants, https://www.youtube.com/watch?v=jwGpEdBpl7o— Iz Harris has some beautiful short film-style poems and essays about her experiences with her own mental illnesses.

Other resources:

Klinic Community Health

www.klinic.mb.ca

Canadian Mental Health Association

www.cmha.ca

Suicide Prevention Resources

www.suicideprevention.ca

The Trevor Project – Resources for LGBTQ2IA+

www.thetrevorproject.org

Resources for LGBT Youth

www.cdc.gov/lgbthealth/youth-resources.htm

Strongest Families Institute

www.strongestfamilies.com

acknowledgments

Thank you to my family, who gets the privilege of seeing the ugliest parts of me that no one else gets to see. But, you still love me and have supported me every step of the way. You're my favourite part of life.

Thank you to my grandparents, who inadvertently inspired my life's purpose and continue to influence my values and worldview.

Thank you to all of my collaborators on this project. This would not be a book if not for all my incredibly talented friends. Thank you to my incredible editor, Kyla Neufeld, for your detailed eye. Thank you to my beta readers, Erin Toews, Tavia McKinnon, Jenny Kelson, and Emily Stobbe-Wiebe. You are all smarter than me. Thank you to all of my social media followers and everyone who has liked or commented on one of my pieces posted there. Thank you to Ariel Gordon, Donna Besel, and Amber O'Reilly, and many other writers I've met on this path to publication, who have been amazingly encouraging of my writing career. I hope eventually I can pass on the gifts and mentorship you gave me.

And last but not at all least, thank you to Amber Wallin. It has been a joy to collaborate with you for the past two years on this book, and get to know you better in the process. I hope you see this book as yours as much as mine.

Thank you to all of the friends who inspired these pieces and me to keep living: Su Jin Kim, Su Hyun Kim, Christina Cooper, Emily Casselman, Megan Pries, Tavia McKinnon, Derek Manaigre, Nicholas Friesen, Sabrina Janke, Brett Hampton, Salma Sedigh, Melissa Taplin, Stacey Liang, Cherise Williams, Amelia Warkentin, Amanda Dueck, and all of the friends I'm still just beginning to love.

Also thank you to all of the members of Incantatem Singers, and my D&D group: Riley Sherlock, Amber Wallin, Nickolas Wiebe, Liliana Nairn, and Erin Toews.

I love you all. This book is for you.

about the author

Alyssa Sherlock has had an overactive imagination since she was a child, and has been a writer most of her life as a result. She's interested in making sense of the world through story, particularly through exploring topics of loneliness, mental health, family, and friendship. She makes her home in the beautiful prairie landscape of Winnipeg, Manitoba.

You can find her writing love letters on her Instagram or Facebook page, @asherlockwrites. You can find more information about Alyssa on her website www.alyssasherlock.com, where you can also sign up for her newsletter to keep up to date on her writing projects.

www.ingramcontent.com/pod-product-compliance
Lightning Source LLC
Chambersburg PA
CBHW040510110526
44587CB00045B/4213